Amel DJERBAL
Nabila BENAMROUCHE
Karim MESKOURI

THE DIABETIC FOOT

Amel DJERBAL
Nabila BENAMROUCHE
Karim MESKOURI

THE DIABETIC FOOT

PATHOPHYSIOLOGY, BACTERIOLOGY, DIAGNOSIS AND MANAGEMENT

ScienciaScripts

Imprint

Any brand names and product names mentioned in this book are subject to trademark, brand or patent protection and are trademarks or registered trademarks of their respective holders. The use of brand names, product names, common names, trade names, product descriptions etc. even without a particular marking in this work is in no way to be construed to mean that such names may be regarded as unrestricted in respect of trademark and brand protection legislation and could thus be used by anyone.

Cover image: www.ingimage.com

This book is a translation from the original published under ISBN 978-620-6-71016-5.

Publisher:
Sciencia Scripts
is a trademark of
Dodo Books Indian Ocean Ltd. and OmniScriptum S.R.L publishing group

120 High Road, East Finchley, London, N2 9ED, United Kingdom
Str. Armeneasca 28/1, office 1, Chisinau MD-2012, Republic of Moldova, Europe
Printed at: see last page
ISBN: 978-620-7-53038-0

THE DIABETIC FOOT: PATHOPHYSIOLOGY, BACTERIOLOGY, DIAGNOSIS AND MANAGEMENT

AMEL DJERBAL, NABILA BENAMROUCHE

KARIM MESKOURI

TABLE OF CONTENTS

I.INTRODUCTION

Because of its burden of morbidity and mortality, diabetes is a global public health problem and a heavy economic and social burden. According to statistics from the International Diabetes Federation (IDF), 4.2 million people with diabetes died in 2019. Today, diabetes is a pandemic affecting more than 425 million people, and this figure is rising every year. In Algeria, prevalence is estimated at 14.4%, giving a total of more than 4.5 million diabetics. If we take into account the margin for improvement announced by the IDF, which is 96%, this rate is likely to double by 2045, meaning that there will be almost 9 million diabetics in Algeria within 20 years [1]. Between 2003 and 2017, Algeria recorded an increase of 80%. The profile of diabetes varies considerably depending on a country's economic situation. In developed countries, the majority of people with diabetes are over 60, whereas in developing countries, most people with diabetes are of working age, between 40 and 60. This difference is likely to continue to exist in 2030, although to a lesser extent, as the average age of people in developing countries will increase slightly more than in developed countries [2].

Apart from acute metabolic complications, diabetes leads to chronic complications linked to vascular damage and secondary neuropathy, affecting three main areas: the eyes, kidneys and feet. The management of diabetic foot lesions has long been neglected. These foot lesions are dominated by ulcers (almost 25% of patients develop an ulcer in the course of their lives), which can become secondarily infected in 40 to 80% of cases, significantly increasing patient morbidity and mortality[3].In addition, these ulcers can be which may or may not be associated with osteitis and may require amputation. Charcot foot lesions are much rarer [2].

II.GENERAL INFORMATION AND REMINDERS

The foot is the most distal part of the lower limb, articulating with the leg bones via the ankle. It is characterised by its different morphotypes and anatomical variations, and provides postural support by bearing the entire weight of the body and ensuring stable support on the ground, as well as locomotion thanks to the mobility of the joints and the rolling of the arch of the foot. It therefore plays an essential role in balance, shock absorption and propulsion. The foot is considered to be a peripheral heart. It acts as a pump to return blood to the heart. The sole of the foot contains a multitude of nerve endings. The foot is made up of 28 bones, 16 joints, 107 ligaments that hold the joints together and 20 intrinsic muscles **[4].**

1.Osteology of the foot

The skeleton of the instep is formed by the lower end of the tibia and fibula, joined by the lower tibio-peroneal joint forming a mortise to which the talus is attached. (Figure 1)
There are 3 groups of bones in the foot:

- The tarsus is made up of seven short bones. It alone represents the upper half of the foot skeleton and widens from back to front from the posterior tarsus to the anterior tarsus.
- The metatarsals

- The phalanges

The last 2 represent the forefoot.

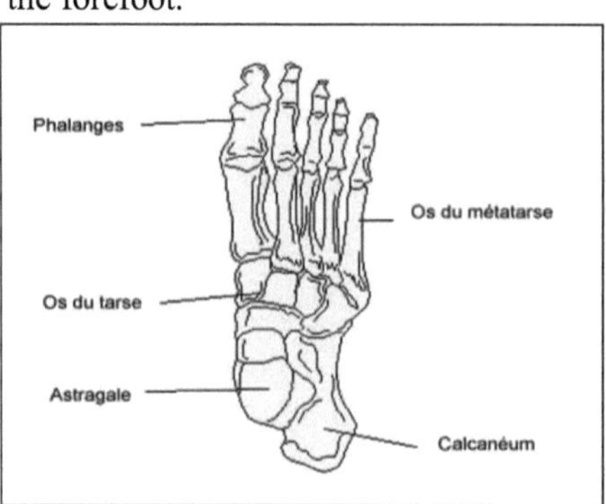

Figure 1. The different bony parts of the foot [4].

1.1. Hind tarsus

It is formed by two superimposed bones: the talus and the calcaneus (Figure 2).

1.1.1. Astragale (Talus)

It is a short, cuboidal bone, elongated in the antero-posterior direction, placed above the arch of the foot, firmly enclosed between the tibio-peroneal mortise, the calcaneum and the scaphoid. It comprises three parts: the body, the neck and the head.

1.1.2. Calcaneum (Calcaneus)

It is the largest of the tarsal bones and forms the posteroinferior part of the tarsus, below the talus. Morphologically, it is divided into three portions:
- **The body:** which forms the skeleton of the heel

- **The greater apophysis**: articulates anteriorly with the ulna

- **The small apophysis**: overhangs the calcaneal groove at the top and front

1.2. Anterior tarsus

Comprising five juxtaposed bones:

- **The ulna**, located on the outer 1/3 of the body
The inner 2/3 are :

- **The three cuneiform bones** (in front)

- **The scaphoid** or navicular bone (at the back), located between the head of the talus and the three cuneiforms. There are four faces (anterior, posterior, superior and inferior) and two extremities (medial and lateral) (Figure 3).

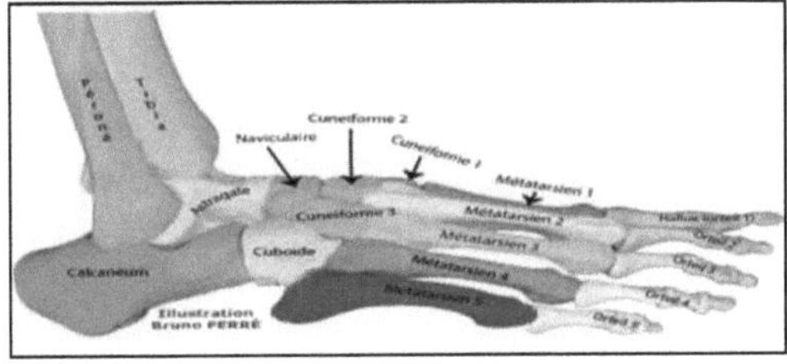

Figure 2. The bones of the foot seen in external profile [4].

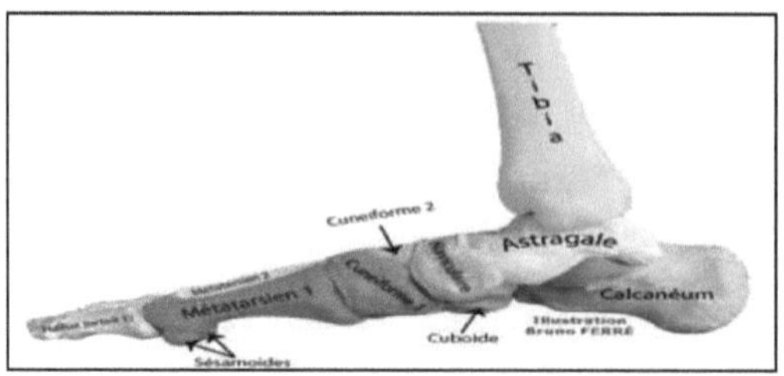

Figure 3. The bones of the foot seen in internal profile [4].

1.3. Foot joints

- The tibio-tarsal joint, which joins the leg to the foot, is a joint that involves three bones: the tibia, the fibula and the talus (Figure 4).
- The astragalo-calcaneal or subtalar joint.

- The medio-tarsal joint (Chopart's joint): this joins the posterior tarsus to the anterior tarsus, and is anatomically made up of two separate joints: the astragalo-scaphoid (or talo-navicular) joint medially and the calcaneo-cuboid joint laterally.
- The tarsometatarsal joint (Lisfranc joint) between the midfoot and forefoot, which corresponds to :
- The first metatarsal and the first cuneiform ;

- The second metatarsal and the second cuneiform.

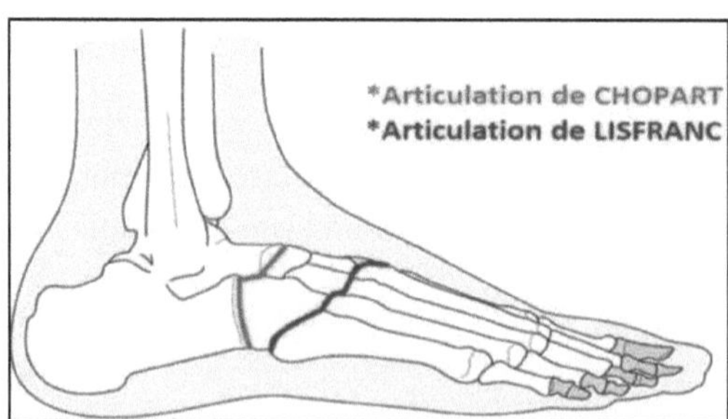

Figure 4: Diagram illustrating the CHOPART and LISFRANC joints [4].

2.Myology of the foot

The intrinsic muscles of the foot are divided into several compartments: plantar, medial, central and lateral, interosseous and dorsal:
- The medial plantar compartment comprises two muscles: the adductor pollicis brevis and the flexor hallucis brevis;
- The central plantar compartment contains seven muscles: the flexor pollicis brevis, the four lumbrici, the flexor digitorum accessory and the adductor hallucis;
- The lateral plantar compartment contains two muscles: the abductor and the flexor pollicis brevis of the fifth toe;
- The interosseous space contains the four plantar interosseous bones and the three dorsal interosseous bones;
- The dorsal compartment contains a single muscle: the extensor digitorum brevis.

3.Innervation of the foot

The nerves of the foot are essentially derived from the sciatic nerve in the thigh. These are branches of the tibial nerve on the one hand, and of the superficial and deep fibular nerves on the other, derived from the common fibular nerve in the leg. A small part of the innervation is provided by branches of the saphenous nerve, derived from the femoral nerve in the thigh.

4.Vascularisation of the foot

The anterior tibial artery becomes the pedal artery and runs along the dorsal surface of the foot.
It gives a dorsal arterial arch which gives (Figure 5) :

- The branch for the 1st interosseous space which anastomoses with the plantar arterial arch;
- Branches for the interosseous spaces.

The posterior tibial artery crosses the malleolus from posterior to anterior and divides into 2 branches in the medial calcaneal canal (Figure 6):
- Medial plantar artery ;

- Lateral plantar artery which forms the plantar arterial arch and gives rise to the plantar intermetacarpal arteries which anastomose with the dorsal arch originating from the dorsal artery of the foot (pedal artery).

A network of anastomoses in the foot to allow bypass surgery for arterial obliteration.

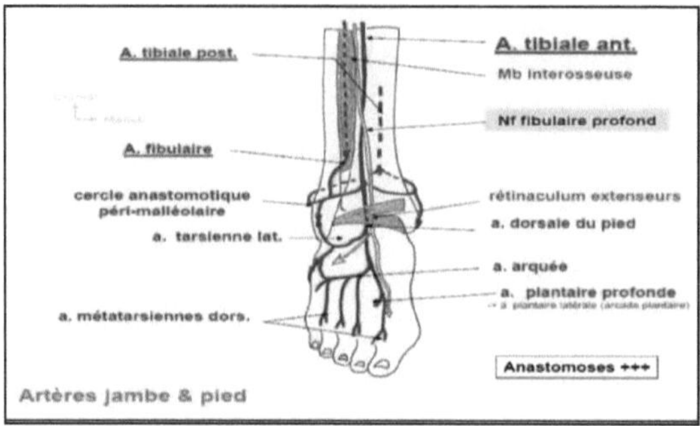

Figure 5. Vascularisation and innervation of the foot - dorsal view [4]

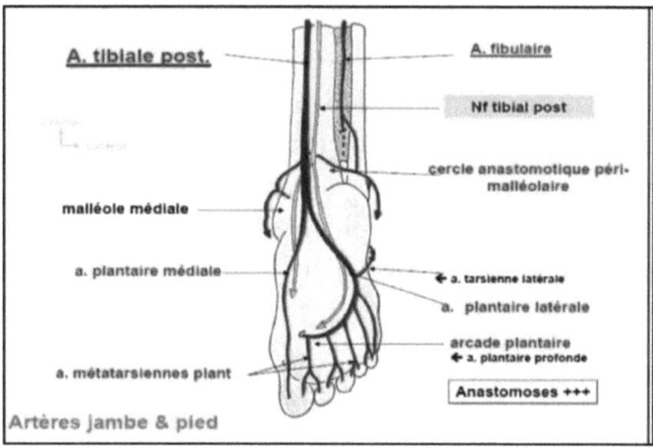

Figure 6. Vascularisation and innervation of the foot - Plantar view [4]

5.Pathways to foot ulceration in people with diabetes

Ulcerations are linked to neuropathy and arteriopathy, which is the prognostic factor for healing; infection is an aggravating factor and increases the risk of amputation. At-risk feet should be screened. Ulcer classifications are essential for defining treatment strategies and providing a prognosis. Before any therapeutic decision is taken, the patient's condition should be assessed clinically and by means of additional tests. neuropathy, vascular insufficiency and infection. Despite the recommendations of the International Consensus on the Diabetic Foot, the organisation of care for diabetic feet remains highly heterogeneous in the different countries of the world; very few have set up centres of reference. The treatment of diabetic feet is multidisciplinary but, as has been shown, the orthopaedic surgeon should play a central role in order to reason in biomechanical terms and avoid recurrences. Although the evidence that foot care education reduces the risk of first ulceration is weak[5] a thorough understanding of the aetiopathogenesis of ulceration is essential if we are to succeed in reducing the incidence of foot lesions and ultimately amputations.

Complications of the diabetic foot are frequent, complex and costly. Demographic trends suggest that these complications, including ulcers, infections, arteriopathy and amputations, will continue to be widespread [6]. The annual incidence of foot ulcers in diabetes is around 2% in most developed countries. Foot ulcers are a frequent complication in diabetic patients. These ulcers are frequently infected and the spread of infection to soft tissue and bony structures is a major causative factor in lower limb amputation [7].

At least half of all amputations occur in people with diabetes, most commonly as a result of an infected diabetic foot ulcer. In the UK, people with diabetes account for over 40% of hospital admissions for major amputations and 73% of emergency admissions for minor amputations [8]. Given that most diabetes-related amputations are preceded by foot ulceration, a A thorough understanding of the causes and management of ulceration is essential to reduce the risk of lower limb amputation. Although the risk of foot ulcers until recently was generally estimated at between 15 and 25%, recent studies suggest that this figure may be as high as 34% [9].

According to Elliott P. Joslin, a renowned diabetologist, "foot ulceration is not an inevitable consequence of diabetes"; rather, ulcers develop as a result of an interaction between specific pathologies of the lower limbs and environmental risks [8].

The Scottish poet Thomas Campbell wrote: "future events cast their shadows before". Although he wasn't talking about foot ulcers at the time, these words can be usefully applied to the deterioration of the diabetic foot [8]. Ulcers do not occur spontaneously, but rather as a result of a combination of factors. Screening the diabetic population for feet at risk of ulceration is the key to preventing diabetic foot complications.

It is increasingly recognised that recurrence of a foot ulcer is common, occurring in up to 50% of cases, and the use of the term "in remission" has been deemed more appropriate than describing an ulcer as "healed". The aim is not necessarily to prevent all wounds, but to maximise ulcer-free, hospital-free and activity-rich days by making each wound recurrence as simple as possible [10, 11].

A study carried out by the Diabetes Amputation Research Group of the Chinese Diabetes Society revealed that, compared with non-diabetic patients, hospital stays were significantly longer (33.5 days compared with 22.0 days) and more expensive ($5932 compared with $4101) for diabetic patients [12]. It is estimated that the medical cost of treating diabetes in China will rise from the current \$4.9 billion to more than \$7.4 billion in 2030. Based on t h e assumption that foot ulcers account for 20% of costs This would impose an economic burden on society [13].

For more than 20 years, a number of countries (United States, Sweden, Netherlands, Belgium, Japan, Switzerland, etc.) have been developing education programmes specifically focused on the diabetic foot, aimed at patients and carers. These countries have gradually set up multidisciplinary foot centres to reduce the number of amputations. In 1995, the Saint-Vincent Declaration [World Health Organisation (WHO)][14] **set the** target of reducing the number of amputations by 50% by the year 2000. In 1996, a group of 15 international experts created the International Working Group on The Diabetic Foot (IWGDF), which published the first International Consensus on the Diabetic Foot in 1999. The International Working Group on the Diabetic Foot (IWGDF) produced recommendations on the prevention and management of diabetic foot disease. In 2019, all the recommendations have been updated, based on systematic literature reviews and the recommendations of multidisciplinary experts from around the world. In 1999, at the 4ème Congress of EFORT (European Federation of National Associations of Orthopaedics and Traumatology), the round table devoted to the diabetic foot reviewed the organisation of diabetic foot care in Europe with a representative from each country. In France, in the absence of an established structure, infected or necrotic lesions of the diabetic foot were treated on an ad hoc basis (amputations, flattening, etc.) in medical-surgical emergency departments by general surgeons, sometimes by vascular surgeons, rarely by orthopaedic surgeons [15]. This round table emphasised the role of the orthopaedic surgeon in the multidisciplinary management of these injuries. Their expertise in joint biomechanics and in the management of these injuries is essential. static disorders and neurogenic osteoarthropathies make it an ideal partner.

IV.PATHOPHYSIOLOGY

Diabetic ulcers have three distinct but interrelated main etiological factors: neuropathy and arteriopathy are two causes secondary to diabetes, and infection is a decompensating factor. Neuropathic and arteriopathic complications rarely occur in isolation, but are generally associated to varying degrees, forming a neuro-ischaemic foot that may develop ulcers. Peripheral ischaemia is a major prognostic factor in the development of ulcers. Infection greatly increases the risk of amputation.

1.Peripheral neuropathy

The exact prevalence of diabetic neuropathy is estimated at between 20 and 60%, depending on the diagnostic methods used; it increases with chronic hyperglycaemia, the length of diabetes and age. It is present in over 90% of diabetic foot ulcers. It is a bilateral polyneuritis of the lower limbs, symmetrical, distal and ascending. A distinction is made between sensory, motor and autonomic disorders.

1.1.Sensory neuropathy

Sensory disorders predominate. Clinical signs vary according to the type of nerve fibres affected. The large fibres are involved in tactile (pressure) and deep (vibratory and proprioceptive) sensitivity, while the small fibres are involved in painful and thermal (hot/cold or thermoalgesic) sensitivity. Trauma, often related to wearing inappropriate footwear, and lesions secondary to friction are not perceived and lead to ulcerations that are often diagnosed late because of the absence of pain.

1.2.Motor neuropathy

It is responsible for weakness and atrophy of the intrinsic muscles of the foot, with the formation of claw toes. Secondly, it contributes to the loss of joint mobility, which is also linked to the glycosylation of connective tissue responsible for fibrosis of the joints, soft tissues and skin.

1.3. Vegetative neuropathy

It leads to skin dryness (reduced perspiration) with the appearance of cracks and fissures, which are a gateway to infection; it also encourages hyperkeratosis in response to hyperpressure. It is also responsible for the opening of arteriovenous shunts and the loss of capillary flow regulation: the neuropathic foot is hot, often oedematous, with dilated dorsal veins.

1.4. Consequences

Peripheral neuropathy is the main factor in diabetic atonic ulcers, with a very hyperkeratotic peripheral halo (different from ulcerations linked to arteriopathy) and neurogenic osteoarthropathies (Charcot's foot).

2. Arteriopathy

It is most often associated to a variable degree with neuropathy (neuroischaemic foot), the frequency of isolated ischaemic lesions being low, around 20%.

2.1. Consequences

Diabetic arteriopathy gradually leads to a state of chronic ischaemia, which aggravates foot lesions. The foot is cold, and the skin becomes thin and shiny. Ischaemic ulcers are often the result of minor trauma. Unlike "neuropathic" ulcers, these ulcers have an erythematous halo without hyperkeratosis. Heel pressure sores, associated with decubitus, on arteriopathy is a chronic lesion. with a poor prognosis. Decompensation of this distal arteritis may lead to ischaemia or even gangrene of one or more toes as a result of acute primary distal thrombosis. The necrosis (black toe) may be dry and limited ("dry gangrene"), but it is often the site of an infection that promotes its spread: this is known as "wet gangrene". Infection is a major aggravating factor in any ulceration, and it also favours distal arterial thrombosis, so that an ulcer which is initially neuropathic may subsequently develop into a predominantly ischaemic condition.

3.Infection

Diabetic patients are more prone than the general population to infections, particularly those of the foot:
- A deficit in cellular defence mechanisms increased by hyperglycaemia, capable of altering leucocyte functions (phagocytosis, adhesion, bactericidal activity, chemotaxis), promoting apoptosis and causing haemorheological disturbances responsible for distal vascularisation disorders;
- The deleterious effect of neuropathy and hyperpressure on the wound ;

- Arteriopathy causes hypoxia and is aggravated by the host's hypermetabolism and microbial cellular metabolism;
- The particular anatomy of the foot is divided into several compartments.

Foot infection in diabetics is usually secondary to a cutaneous wound and corresponds to a multiplication of micro-organisms leading to tissue damage, with or without an inflammatory response in the patient. However, like all chronic wounds, these are colonised by low-virulence aerobic and anaerobic bacteria from the cutaneous commensal flora, endogenous flora or the environment. All bacteria, whether commensal or pathogenic, contribute to the chronicity of the infection. Infection must therefore be distinguished from bacterial colonisation. The diagnosis of foot infection in diabetics is clinical, not microbiological: it is based on clinical data proposed by the International Working Group on the Diabetic Foot (IWGDF).
Infection is defined by the presence of at least two inflammatory manifestations: enlargement, induration, peri-lesional erythema, local tenderness or pain, local warmth, presence of pus.
The classification of foot wound infection is divided into four grades:

- Grade 1: colonisation without local signs ;

- Grade 2: moderate localised superficial infection, skin involvement only ;
- Grade 3: deep infection, beyond the skin and cutaneous tissue ;

- Grade 4: superficial or deep infection with systemic signs.

Diabetic foot infections are :

- Either superficial (above the aponeurosis) with a picture of acute bacterial dermo-hypodermatitis (DHB), necrotizing or non-necrotizing;
- Or deep, affecting the superficial fascia, muscles or osteoarticular structures, resulting in a variety of symptoms: necrotising fasciitis (FN-DHB), wet

gangrene, abscess, phlegmon, osteitis and osteoarthritis.

Bone infection is a very frequent complication of diabetic foot ulcers. Clinical-biological collaboration is essential in diagnosing the infection and isolating the pathogenic bacteria[16, 17].

All chronic wounds are colonised by bacteria. As a result, the diagnosis of foot wound infection in diabetic patients cannot be based solely on the bacteriological result of a wound sample, but must be assessed clinically. Clinical criteria are used to classify the severity of foot wound infection (Table 1). However, the clinical manifestations used in this classification may be reduced in diabetics. It is therefore quite possible that certain infections may not be diagnosed as severe. are not detected when they are first presented. This delay in initiating appropriate treatment can lead to the infection spreading, potentially threatening the integrity of a lower limb. This progression can be rapid, as it is associated with an environment that favours it. A very large number of bacteria are responsible for foot wound infections. Gram-positive aerobic bacteria are the most common, along with Staphylococcus aureus and β-hemolytic streptococci. This predominance of Gram-positive bacteria is only seen in Western countries. Gram-negative aerobic bacilli, mainly from the Enterobacteriaceae family (Proteus mirabilis, Escherichia coli, Klebsiellaspp.), are generally found in chronic or previously treated infections. Pseudomonas aeruginosa is often isolated after long-term hospitalisation, the application of moist dressings or footbaths. It is the bacterium most frequently isolated in developing countries (particularly South-East Asia). However, its pathogenic role is debatable. Finally, strict anaerobic bacteria, most often gram-positive cocci but also gram-negative bacilli, are often associated with aerobic bacteria [17].The bacterial ecology of osteitis, which differs from material osteitis, is shown in table 2. Superficial infections are usually monomicrobial (staphylococcus aureus, streptococcus, etc.), whereas deep infections are polymicrobial (Gram-positive, Gram-positive and anaerobic bacteria). Samples taken during consultations, even under strict conditions, have a value that needs to be put into perspective before appropriate antibiotic therapy is introduced. In 2001, in a study of 44 cases of osteitis in diabetic patients undergoing surgical treatment [18], a comparison was made between preoperative bacteriology and bacteriology of deep soft tissue and bone tissue carried out during the operation. Culture results were inconsistent in 46% of cases, partially concordant in 26% and totally concordant in only 24% of cases. Repeated preoperative bacteriological samples taken by trained professionals were monobacterial in 76% of cases.

Table 1. PEDIS (Perfusion - Extend - Depth - Infection - Sensation) classification [41].

Perfusion (vascularisation)	
Grade P1	Pas de symptômes, pas de signes d'artériopathie périphérique (ABI : 0,9–1,1 ou $TcPO_2$ > 60 mm Hg)
Grade P2	Symptômes ou signes d'artériopathie périphérique mais pas d'ischémie critique du membre
Grade P3	Ischémie critique du membre ($TcPO_2$ < 30 mm Hg ou pression systolique de cheville < 50 mm Hg)
Extend (étendue)	
	Taille de la plaie mesurée en cm^2 après débridement
Depth (profondeur)	
Grade D1	Ulcère superficiel limité au derme
Grade D2	Ulcère profond, pénétrant sous le derme jusqu'aux structures sous-cutanées, impliquant les fascias, les muscles ou les tendons
Grade D3	Toutes les couches suivantes, y compris l'os et/ou l'articulation (contact osseux ou ulcère pénétrant jusqu'à l'os)
Infection (infection)	
Grade I1	Aucun symptôme ni signe d'infection
Grade I2	Infection impliquant la peau et les tissus sous-cutanés (au moins 2 des critères suivants : œdème local ou induration, érythème > 0,5–2 cm, douleur à la pression, chaleur locale, écoulement purulent)
Grade I3	Érythème > 2 cm plus un des critères ci-dessus (œdème, douleur à la pression, chaleur, écoulement) ou infection plus profonde (abcès, ostéomyélite, arthrite septique, fasciite…)
Grade I4	Infection avec signes systémiques (au moins 2 des critères suivants : température > 38 °C ou < 36 °C, fréquence cardiaque < 90/min, fréquence respiratoire > 20/min, $PaCO_2$ < 32 mm Hg, globules blancs > 12 000, 10 % formes leucocytaires indifférenciées)
Sensation (sensibilité)	
Grade S1	Aucune perte de la sensibilité de protection
Grade S2	Perte de la sensibilité de protection

Table 2. Ecology of osteitis in diabetic foot wounds [17].

Bacteria/ References	Whe at et al, 1986 , Arch Inter n Med	Newm an et al, 1991, JAMA	Lave ry et al, 1995, J Foot Ankl e Surg	Sennev i lle et al., 2006, Clin Infect Dis	Aragon- Sanchez et al, 2008, Diabetol o gia	Arago n- Sanch ez et al., 2010, Diabe t ic foot Ankle	Maliz os et al., 2010, Injur y	Lesens et al., 2011, Clin Microb i al Infect	Elamuru g an et al, 2011, Int J Surg
Gram-positive cocci (%)									
S. aureus	40	31	47	26	47	38	86	33	31
SCN	10	50	11	26	11	12	10	14	-
Streptococ ci	45	27	61	12	3	1	-	9	3
Enterococc uss pp.	30	8	28	8	1	-	18	12	-
Other	10	-	-	2	-	-	-	4	2
Gram-negative bacilli (%)									
Enterobact eria s	55	20	14	18	29	36	11	18	32
Pseudomo nass pp.	5	15	11	2	9	10	43	2	19
Acinetobac ter spp.	-	-	-	-	-	3	-	-	13
Anaerobes	60	4	15	5	-	-	-	4	-
Polymicro bial	70	ND	83	ND	ND	ND	ND	ND	ND

ND: not determined; SCN: coagulase-negative staphylococci.

4."Biomechanics of ulceration

It is the combination of diabetic neuropathy and plantar hyperpressure that is responsible for the majority of ulcerations in diabetics. Patients without neuropathy who have high plantar pressure for various reasons (degenerative or even inflammatory foot deformities, as in rheumatoid arthritis, etc.) rarely develop ulcers, as they adapt their gait to the pain caused by the hyperpressure. The loss of sensitivity to pressure and pain is responsible for the repetition of a This is caused by localised hyper-pressure and shearing forces on the area of hy-perkeratosis, under which a collection develops, eventually leading to the formation of an ulcer. In addition, any mechanical, thermal or chemical injury may also be responsible for ulceration, which is diagnosed late because of the absence of pain (Figure 7).

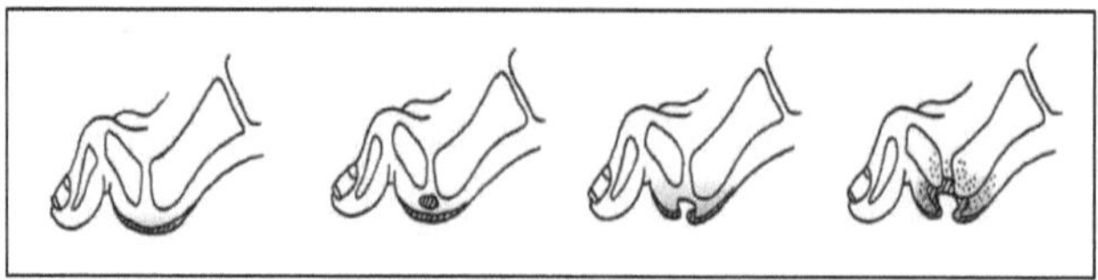

Figure 7. Mechanism of ulcer developing from repetitive or excessive mechanical hyperpressure [39].

4.1. Plantar pressure threshold

Most ulcerations occur on the little toes, the hallux and opposite the metatarsal heads. These areas have been studied in an attempt to find a predictive threshold for ulceration. Figures of 5 to 10 kg/cm2 have been put forward **[19, 20].** Armstrong reports a pressure threshold of 7 kg/cm2 (700 kPa) as identifying patients at risk of ulceration, but with a sensitivity of only 70% and a specificity of 65%. These values vary depending on the patient, the anatomical area and the technical conditions of the study. In addition, this threshold is probably linked to the duration of exposure: the longer the patient walks, the lower the threshold should be (Figure 8).

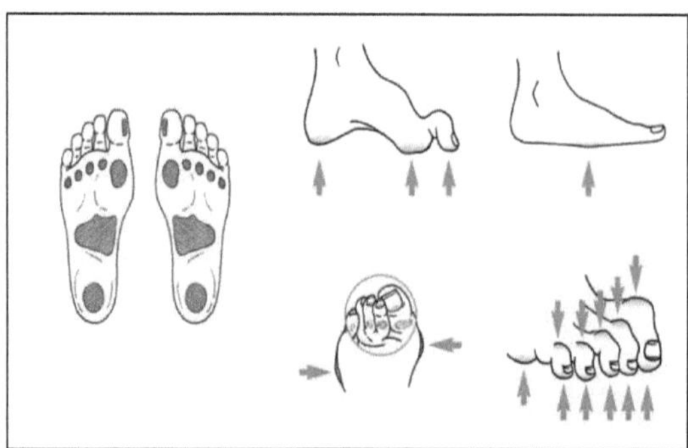

Figure 8: Areas of the foot most at risk of ulceration [39].

4.2. Factors in plantar hyperpressure and ulceration

Hyper-pressure when walking and ulcerations are the result of several factors.

4.2.1. Factors intrinsic to the foot

The morphology of the foot can predispose to plantar hyperpressures, without being related to diabetes: hollow foot, hallux valgus, anomalies in metatarsal length (Greek foot, long second metatarsal), etc. Toe claws are very common in neuropathic diabetics. Plantar calluses and corns secondary to deformities behave like a foreign body, causing localised hyperpressure. The reduced range of motion of the ankle, subtalar and first metatarsophalangeal joints found in diabetics transfers pressure to the forefoot when walking. Finally, severe deformities of the foot secondary to osteoarticular destruction (Charcot foot) are a source of hyperpressure, in particular the "blotting pad" appearance of the foot, responsible for ulcers under the midfoot.

4.2.2. Extrinsic factors

Unsuitable footwear (too narrow at the toe, too tight, lack of cushioning, prominent seams, etc.) is thought to be responsible for more than 40% of ulcers. A foreign body (stone, nail, drawing pin, etc.) that has gone unnoticed in the shoe can sometimes be the cause. Ulcers can be prevented primarily by adapting footwear and checking the contents of shoes before putting them on. Obesity is traditionally considered to be a factor that increases plantar pressure.

4.2.3. Behavioural factors

Barefoot walking is one of the main causes of sole ulceration. The visual problems associated with retinopathy can make it impossible to monitor the feet and care for the nails on a daily basis. Prevention through education must therefore be aimed not only at the patient, but also at his or her family, paramedical and medical entourage. The feet of diabetics should be examined daily by the patient and those around him, and systematically at the time of any medical consultation. Regular pedicure, including nail care and careful removal of hyperkeratosis (calluses, corns), is an essential part of prevention.

4.2.4. Iatrogenic factors

Inappropriate nail care or pedicure (use of coricides) can cause wounds. Amputation of the first ray is serious from a functional point of view, as normal propulsion at the end of the stance phase is lost and stresses under the metatarsal heads and lateral toes increase, leading to the formation of claws [21]. This leads to more than 70% of repeat surgeries for ulcer recurrence on the lateral radii. Similarly, the resection of a metatarsal head increases the pressure under the adjacent head [22].Finally, the progressive "sausage-making" of the toes of the forefoot leads to recurrences and regular repeat surgery; thus leaving two or three medial toes... on a forefoot is a mechanical aberration which can only lead to a rapid recurrence of ulcers.

4.3. Feet at risk

It is essential to classify at-risk feet in order t o   develop prevention strategies. Depending on the complication rate, the IWGDF has proposed classifying diabetic feet into four risk groups [23]: **Group 0: (very low risk):** absence of neuropathy and arteriopathy **Group 1: (low risk):** presence of neuropathy or arteriopathy **Group 2: (moderate risk):** neuropathy + arteriopathy or neuropathy associated with à of deformities or arteriopathy associated à   one deformities **Group 3 (severe risk):** neuropathy or arteriopathy and one or more of the following:
-History of foot ulcers ;

-Lower limb amputation (minor or major);

-End stage renal disease.

This classification is used in Belgium in the diabetes passport and to determine reimbursement for chiropody care. A French multicentre study [24] investigated the prevalence of risk factors for foot ulceration by conducting a one-day survey of all diabetics seen in hospital or in consultation in 16 French diabetes centres. Of 664 patients, 15.8% had ulceration. Of the 555 evaluable patients without ulceration, 7.2% had a history of ulceration or amputation, 27.1% had neuropathy (monofilament), 17% had arteriopathy of the lower limbs, and 21.1% had orthopaedic deformities. According to the IWGDF classification, 17.5% of patients were at high risk (groups 2 and 3), which justifies the implementation of a real screening and prevention policy.

4.3.1.Classification of ulcers

The classification of ulcers is of vital importance in daily practice. It helps in communication between healthcare professionals, in assessing prognosis and choosing the best therapeutic strategy, and in auditing clinical results between units and populations.

Monteiro-Soares et al [25] found a large number of proposed classification and scoring systems for diabetic foot ulcers, suggesting that none are ideal for routine use in populations worldwide. This may also reflect the differing purposes of classification and scoring systems for communication between healthcare professionals (irrespective of the level of clinical care), for clinical prognosis and treatment guidance, and for clinical audit of outcomes across units and populations. From this perspective, a classification system can be defined as a descriptive tool, dividing patients into groups without necessarily linking it to the risk of an adverse outcome. The key factors considered to contribute to the scoring of the classifications are of three types: patient-related (end-stage renal disease), limb-related (peripheral arterial disease and loss of protective tenderness) and ulcer-related (surface, depth, site, single or multiple and infection). A consensus was then reached [26, 27], based on expert opinion and the eight factors that were consistently and significantly related to ulcer outcomes that would ideally form the basis of a classification system:

- Patient factors: end-stage renal disease ;

- Limb factors: peripheral arterial disease; loss of protective sensitivity;
- Ulcer factors: area; depth; location (forefoot / hindfoot); number (single / multiple); infection.

By consensus, the following five clinical scenarios were defined as being the most frequently encountered and requiring classification of foot ulcers in diabetic patients:
- Communication between healthcare professionals on the characteristics of an ulcer ;
- To assess an individual's prognosis in relation to the outcome of their ulcer;
- To guide management in the specific clinical scenario of a patient with an infected ulcer;
- To help decide whether a patient with an ulcer would benefit from lower limb revascularisation;
- Support regional/national/international auditing to enable comparison between institutions.

For each clinical scenario, a clinical question was formulated taking into account the PICO elements: population, intervention, comparator and outcome. We recommend: **(i)** for communication between healthcare professionals, the use of the SINBAD system (which includes site, ischaemia, neuropathy, bacterial infection and depth); **(ii)** noexisting classification to predict the prognosis of an individual ulcer; **(iii)** the InfectiousDiseases Society of America / IWGDF (IDSA / IWGDF) classification for the assessment of infection; **(iv)** the WIfI (wound, ischaemia and foot infection) system for the assessment of perfusion and the likely benefit of revascularisation; and **(v)** the SINBAD classification for the verification of population outcomes.

4.3.1.1. In a person with diabetes and a foot ulcer, use the SINBAD system to communicate with healthcare professionals about the characteristics of the ulcer.

The SINBAD system is quick and easy to use, requiring no specialised equipment beyond the clinical examination alone, and contains the following features information needed to enable triage by a specialist team. It would therefore be possible to use this classification system in locations where such facilities, including non-invasive perfusion measurements, are not readily available, which is the case for the majority of geographical settings where diabetic foot ulcers occur. If used for communication between healthcare professionals, it is important to use the individual clinical descriptors and not simply the total score. This classification has been validated for ulcer healing and amputation prediction, **[28-33]** with good results and reliability **[34, 35]** (Table 3).

Table 3. SINBAD system [39]

Category	Definition	Score
Website	Forefoot	0
	Mid and hind foot	1
Ischemia	Intact pedal artery blood flow: at least one pulse palpable	0
	Clinical evidence of reduced pedal flow	1
Neuropathy	Protective sensation intact	0
	Lost sense of protection	1
Infection	No	0
bacterial	Present	1
Zone	Ulcer <1 cm 2	0
	Ulcer ≥ 1 cm 2	1
Depth	Ulcers confined to the skin and subcutaneous tissues	0
	Ulcers affecting the muscle, tendon or deeper areas	1
Total possible score		6

4.3.1.2. Do not use any of the classification / scoring systems currently available to propose an individual prognosis for a person with diabetes and a foot ulcer.

Meggitt-Wagner, PEDIS, SINBAD, University of Texas and WIfI have been externally validated for the prediction of ulcer healing and lower limb amputation within cohorts [25] but not at the individual level. In addition, WIfI has been extensively validated in cohorts of patients with severe limb ischaemia on several continents, with one cohort specific to diabetic foot ulcer and five additional papers including >75% ulcer patients [36, 37].

- Megitt-Wagner classification [38].

This is the oldest and was for a long time the most widely used. It is simple, but it does not include the factors of loss of protective sensitivity, infection and ischaemia, and therefore its usefulness may vary from one country to another.

The University of Texas is a descriptive classification, rather than a scoring system, containing only three of the eight prognostic factors identified by the expert panel [34, 35].

- **PEDIS classification** (Perfusion - Extend - Depth -Infection - Sensation) :
This is the most recent, based on an international consensus. It was developed by the IWGDF and published in 2003 **[39]**.
PEDIS was originally developed as a descriptive classification for use in research and not for prognostic purposes. It does not include patient-related factors (end-stage renal disease) or the location or number of foot ulcers. PEDIS has been validated in two studies both for wound healing and for a composite endpoint of non-healing, amputation and death [30, 40]. It has also been shown to have good reliability **[35],** although it is not a scoring system. This classification is based on the five parameters **[41] that** are important to consider when treating ulcers in diabetics (Table 1):
- "Perfusion (vascularisation): depending on the vascularisation, there are three grades, from P1 (absence of arteriopathy) to P3 (critical ischaemia of the limb);
-"Extend: the size of the wound is measured in square centimetres;

-"Depth: there are three grades, from D1 (limited to the dermis) to D3 (bone involvement);
- "Infection: there are four grades, from I1 (no infection) to I4 (systemic infection);
- "Sensation: there are two grades, S1 (normal sensitivity) and S2 (loss of sensitivity).
Thus, each diabetic wound can be characterised by five elements, and each has a different prognosis.

4.3.1.3. In a diabetic patient with an infected foot ulcer, use the IDSA / IWGDF classification of infections to characterise and guide the management of the infection.

The IWGDF / ISDA classification includes four degrees of severity for diabetic foot infection (table 4). It was originally developed as part of the PEDIS classification for research purposes and is used as a management guide, in particular to identify patients requiring hospitalisation for intravenous antibiotics. Although the components of each grade are complex and a previous study showed only moderate reliability, the criteria are widely used. Unsurprisingly, given the context of the IWGDF / IDSA classification, it is a good predictor of the need for hospitalisation [42]. However, it has also been validated for the risk of both major and minor amputation [31, 34].

Table 4. International Working Group on the Diabetic Foot System (IWGDF)/ Infectious Diseases Society of America (IDSA) [41].

Clinical manifestations	Severity of infection	Grade PEDIS
Wound without pus or inflammation	Not infected	1
Presence of at least 2 signs of inflammation (pus, erythema, tenderness, heat or induration), but any cellulitis/erythema extends over ≤ 2 cm around the ulcer and infection is limited to the skin or superficial subcutaneous tissue; no other local complications or disease systemic	Benin	2
Infection (as above) in a patient who is systemically healthy and metabolically stable but has ≥ 1 of the following features: cellulitis extending> 2 cm, lymphangitic streaks, spread under superficial fascia, deep tissue abscess, gangrene and damage to muscle, tendon, joint or bone	Moderate	3
Infection in a patient with sepsis or metabolic instability (e.g. fever, chills, tachycardia, hypotension, confusion, vomiting, leukocytosis, acidosis, severe hyperglycaemia or azotemia).	Severe	4

4.3.1.4.   In a diabetic person with a foot ulcer who is managed in an environment where appropriate vascular intervention expertise is available, use the WIfI score to aid decision making in assessing perfusion and the likelihood of benefiting from revascularisation.

WIfI (Table 5) uses a combination of scores for wound (based on ulcer depth or extent of gangrene), ischaemia (based on ankle-brachial index (ABI) or $TcPO_2$ and foot infection (based on IWGDF / IDSA criteria) to provide a one-year risk of amputation and a one-year benefit for revascularisation [43]. WIfI requires the use of specialised measures of foot perfusion indices and although it therefore contains most of the key variables to enable the triage of people with DFU, it is not ideal for use in primary/community care (Figure 9). Only two classification systems have been developed that provide stratification that aligns with clinical decision-making: IWGDF/IDSA and WIfI [25]. Of note, although IWGDF/IDSA is incorporated into WIfI, in situations where only infection is being assessed and the equipment is not available to use WIfI, IWGDF/IDSA infection classification can stand alone.

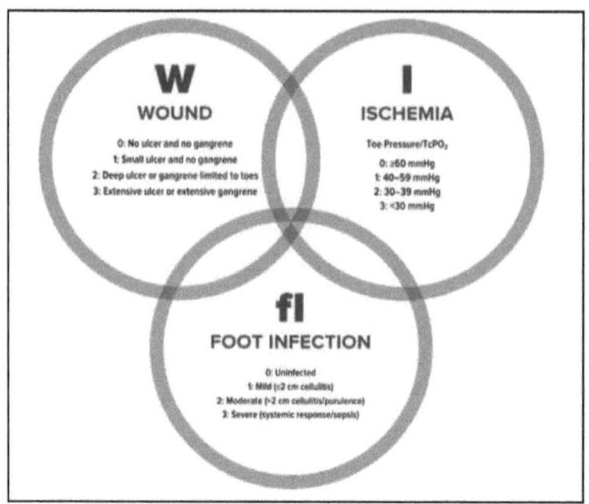

Figure 9. WIfI classification system, TcPO 2, transcutaneous oxygen pressure [25].

Table 5. WIFI foot wound, ischaemia and infection system [25].

Grade 1	• Pas de signe d'infection

Grade 2	• Infection touchant uniquement la peau et le tissu sous-cutané
	• Au moins 2 items suivants:
	  – Œdème ou induration
	  – Rougeur >0,5 cm et <2 cm
	  – Douleur locale
	  – Chaleur locale
	  – Ecoulement purulent

Grade 3	• Rougeur >2 cm, associée à l'un des items suivants: œdème, douleur, chaleur, écoulement Ou • Atteinte des tissus profonds: arthrite septique, ostéomyélite, abcès, fascéite • Pas de signe systémique

Grade 4	• Réponse inflammatoire systémique (SIRS)
	• Présence d'au moins 2 items:
	  – Tachycardie >90 bpm
	  – Tachypnée >20 cycles/min
	  – Température >38°C ou <36°C
	  – PaCO₂ <32 mmHg
	  – Globules blancs >12 000/mm³
	  – 10% de forme immature

4.3.1.5. Use the SINBAD system for any regional/national/international audit to enable inter-institutional comparisons of outcomes for patients with diabetes and foot ulcers.

The term "audit" refers to the characterisation of all DFUs managed in a particular area or centre, in order to compare results with a reference population or national standard, and does not refer to the financial implications of care. At present, SINBAD is the only classification system that meets all these criteria. It has been validated for healing and amputation risk in various populations with diabetic foot ulcers [28, 31, 33, 44, 45] and has been shown to be acceptable to clinicians in the UK National Diabetes Foot Care audit of over 20,000 DFUs [28].

The majority of ulcers are favoured by neuropathy, but it is the neuropathic state that is the most important factor. vascular disease which determines prognosis. Infection is an additional serious factor in the prognosis of the limb and the survival of the patient.

V.DIAGNOSTIC

When faced with a wound in a diabetic patient, all doctors must diagnose neuropathy before taking any therapeutic decision. But it is above all the search for and assessment of vascular insufficiency and infection which will be the decisive prognostic factors. These two elements are also necessary to classify the wound according to the PEDIS system.

Beforehand, the interview will specify :

- Age of diabetes, glycaemic control (glycated haemoglobin level: an Hb A1 C value > 7% indicates poorly controlled diabetes);
-Associated complications, in particular retinopathy and renal failure

-A history of ulcers or minor amputations;

-How the wound that prompted the consultation arose, how long it has been there and what treatment has already been given.

1.Neuropathy

Neuropathy associated with diabetes is progressive but silent. It should therefore be systematically sought during any foot examination in a diabetic patient. The diagnosis of neuropathy in a diabetic patient, even one with no wounds or history of wounds, calls for specific preventive education, as neuropathy is a factor in the development of foot ulcers. Almost all diabetic patients with ulcers have sensory neuropathy; Charcot foot is also a consequence of neuropathy.

1.1.Screening tests: a sensory examination of the foot

Peripheral neuropathy can be detected using a 10 g monofilament (5.07 Semmes-Weinstein) (detects loss of protective sensitivity) and a tuning fork (128 Hz, detects loss of vibratory sensation). This is a simple clinical diagnosis, and the loss of protective sensitivity is assessed by the two simple tests described below.

1.1.1.Monofilament 5.07 of 10 g

Semmens-Weinstein monofilaments are a rapid means of exploring pressure sensitivity. These are Nylon™ threads calibrated so that when applied perpendicularly to the patient's skin, their curvature corresponds to a given force. Several are available, but the 5.07 curve Nylon™ monofilament is generally used, equivalent to a force of 10g corresponding to the level of sensation needed to prevent foot ulceration. In general, several sites on the plantar surface of the foot are explored, three plantar points should be sensitive: the pulp of the hallux, the head of the first and fifth metatarsals. It is recommended that each site be tested three times in succession, including a dummy (yes/no answer) (Table 6). This is the most reliable screening test. Any practitioner treating a diabetic should have one.

How do I take the test?

- First apply the monofilament to the patient's hands (or elbow or forehead) to demonstrate how it feels;
- Test three different sites on both feet, choosing from those illustrated in Figure 10 ;
- Make sure that the patient cannot see if and where the examiner is applying the filament;
- Apply the monofilament perpendicular to the skin surface (Figure 11A) with sufficient force to cause the filament to bend or curl (Figure 11B);
- The total duration of the approach -> skin contact -> and removal of the filament should be approximately 2 seconds;
- Do not apply the filament directly to an ulcer, callus, scar or necrotic tissue;
- Do not allow the filament to slide over the skin or make repetitive contact with the test site;
- Press the filament against the skin and ask the patient if they feel the pressure being applied ("yes"/"no") and then where they feel the pressure (for example, "left foot/right heel);
- Repeat this application twice on the same site, but alternate it with at least one "dummy" application in which no filament is applied (a total of three questions per site);
- Protective sensitivity is present at each site if the patient responds correctly to two out of three applications; absent with two out of three incorrect responses;
- Encourage patients during the test by giving positive feedback.

Monofilaments tend to temporarily lose their buckling strength after being used several times on the same day, or permanently after long-term use. Depending on the type of monofilament, it is suggested that the monofilament should not be used for the next 24 hours after 10 to 15 patients have been assessed and 70 to 90 patients have had the monofilament replaced after use.

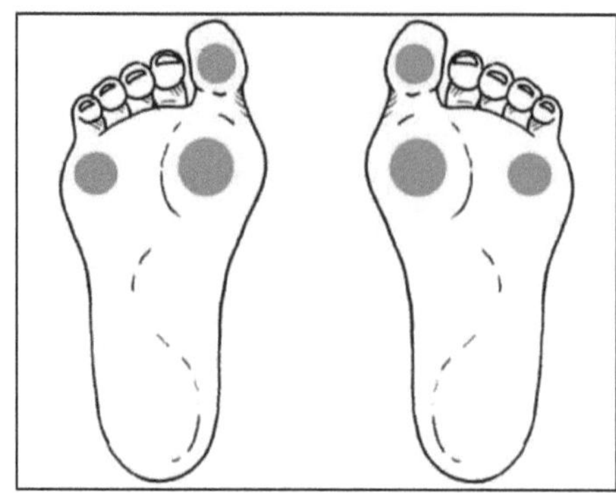

Figure 10. Sites that should be tested for loss of protective sensitivity with Semmes-Weinstein 10 g monofilament [39].

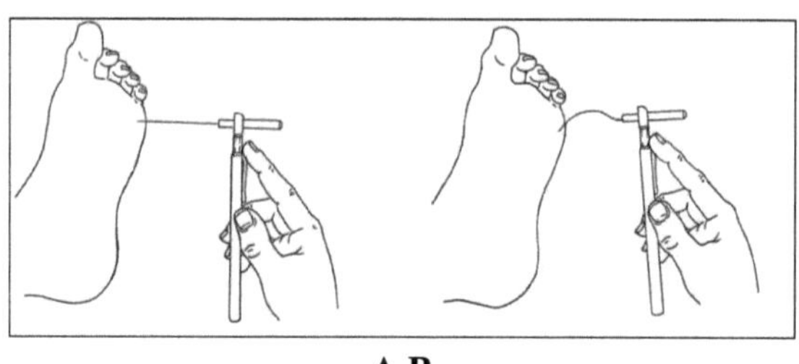

Figure 11. Correct method of using the 10 g monofilamentSemmes-Weinstein [39].

Table 6. Foot screening sheet for clinical examination [39].

Presence of a full-thickness ulcer	Yes/No
Risk factors for foot ulceration	
Peripheral neuropathy (one or more of the following tests) Undetectable protective sensitivity (monofilament) Vibration (128 Hz tuning fork) undetectable Light touch (Ipswich touch test) undetectable	Yes/No Yes/No Yes/No
Foot pulses - Posterior tibial artery absent -Dorsal pedal artery absent	Yes/No Yes/No
Other Foot deformity or excessive bony prominences Limited joint mobility Signs of abnormal pressure such as :	Yes/No Yes/No Yes/No
Rough discolouration on dependence Poor foot hygiene Inappropriate footwear Previous ulcer Lower limb amputation	Yes/No Yes/No Yes/No Yes/No Yes/No

1.1.2. Tuning fork 128 Hz

It explores the vibratory sensitivity of the dorsal surface of the head of the first metatarsal.

-First, apply the tuning fork to the patient's wrist (or elbow or collarbone) to demonstrate how it feels;

-Make sure that the patient cannot see if or where the examiner is applying the tuning fork;

- Apply the tuning fork to a piece of bone on the dorsal side of the distal phalanx of the first toe (or another toe if the hallux is missing);

- Apply the tuning fork perpendicularly, using constant pressure (Figure 12) ;

- Repeat this application t w i c e , but alternate it with at least one "fictitious" application in which the tuning fork does not vibrate;

-The test is positive if the patient answers at least two out of three questions correctly, and negative if two out of three answers are incorrect;

-If the patient is unable to detect vibrations on the toe, repeat the test more proximally (e.g. malleolus, tibial tuberosity);

-Encourage the patient during the test by giving positive feedback.

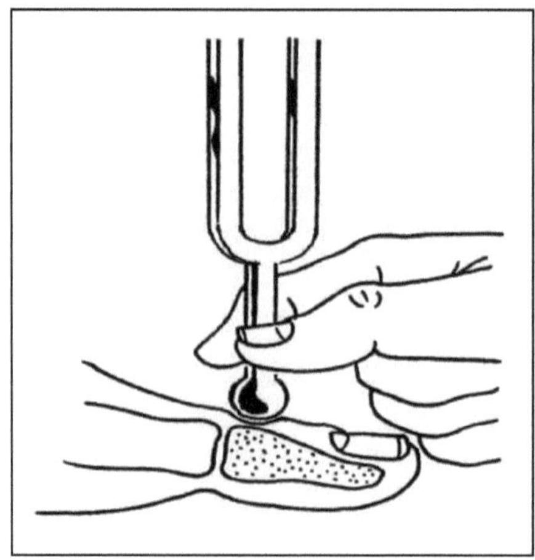

Figure 12: Appropriate method of using a 128 Hz tuning fork to check vibration sensation[39].

1.1.3. Light touch test

This simple test (also known as the Ipswich Touch test) can be used to screen for loss of protective sensitivity when the 10 gram monofilament or 128 HZ tuning fork is not available, but its accuracy in predicting foot ulcers has not been established.

-Explain the procedure and make sure everything is understood;

- Ask the subject to close their eyes and say yes when they feel the touch;
- The examiner lightly touches the tips of the first, third and fifth toes of both feet sequentially with the tip of his index finger / forefinger for 1 to 2 seconds;
-When you touch, don't push, don't touch;

- "LOPS"(Loose Of Protective Sensation) is likely when light touch is not detected in ≥ 2 sites.

1.1.4. New surveillance systems

Efforts to identify pre-ulcer inflammation in the last generation have now led to home monitors that can alert patients up to several weeks before a potential complication[46]. Similarly, smart insoles combined with smart watches may be able to identify potentially damaging pressure, which over time can lead to blistering or callus and tissue loss[47].

2. Vascular insufficiency

Vascular disease must be systematically sought in diabetic feet, as the associated neuropathy usually masks the classic symptoms of vascular insufficiency, particularly pain. The clinical examination can be misleading. Pallor and coldness of the skin, classic signs, are often absent due to vegetative neuropathy associated with the diabetic foot. Because of mediacalcosis, the presence of a pedal and posterior tibial pulse does not mean that there are no microangiopathic lesions. It is therefore necessary to systematically perform a venous filling test.

2.1. Non-invasive diagnostic tests

They are essential for assessing the arterial quality of the lower limbs in diabetics.

2.1.1. Ankle/arm systolic pressure index

The ankle-brachial index (ABI) is a quick and easy way of detecting arterial disease of the lower limbs. The systolic pressure (in millimetres of mercury) of both arms, both pedal arteries and the posterior tibial arteries is measured using a continuous-flow pocket Doppler device.The ICB is the ratio between the highest pressure at the ankles and the highest pressure at the arm:

- ICB > 1: inconclusive value, linked to mediacalcosis (calcification of the media) and does not allow arterial insufficiency to be ruled out;
-ICB = 0.9-1.1: normal value ;

- ICB = 0.5-0.9 (ankle pressure > 50 mm Hg): vascular damage; patient asymptomatic or with claudication;
-BCI < 0.5 (systolic ankle pressure < 50 mm Hg): critical ischaemia.

2.1.2. Measurement of TcPO2

Transcutaneous measurement of the dorsum of the foot reflects local arterial flow and skin oxygenation. It requires expensive equipment (a specially developed polarographic electrode) and takes a relatively long time to perform (30 to 45 minutes). Measurement of TcPO2 is reproducible and is not influenced by mediacalcosis, but must be carried out under standardised conditions (ambient temperature, resting situation, etc.). TcPO2 is read after a state of equilibrium has been reached (15 to 20 min) on a supine patient, with the electrode placed on the back of the foot:

-TcPO2 > 60 mm Hg: normal vascularisation;

- TcPO2 = 30-60 mm Hg: sign of vascular damage but not of critical ischaemia;
-TcPO2 < 30 mm Hg: critical ischaemia.

The measurement of TcPO2 has a prognostic value for wound healing: a value of less than 30 mm Hg is generally accepted as the threshold value for achieving wound healing, with the wound healing rate falling below 30% of cases. Below 10 mm Hg, the prognosis is poor in the short term. It should be noted that TcPO2 is falsely lowered in cases of inflammatory or infectious oedema of the dorsum of the foot.

It can also be measured with the leg dangling. Staged measurement of TcPO2 can help, in conjunction with the practitioner's clinical experience, to determine the level of amputation.

2.1.3. Medical vascular imaging

However, non-invasive methods are insufficient to assess arterial damage, and various vascular imaging investigations may be necessary.

2.1.3.1. Echo-Doppler

This is the most appropriate diagnostic test for screening for diabetic arteriopathy. It is performed regularly as part of the endocrinological work-up for diabetics. It assesses the patency of the distal aorta and the iliac, femoropopliteal and infrapopliteal arteries. Mediacalcosis limits visualisation of the arterial lumen of the infrapopliteal stage, but analysis of the velocities of the peripheral arteries makes it possible to isolate segmental stenoses or obliterations. This non-invasive test can also be used to determine the BCI.

2.1.3.2. Angio-MRI

It is currently playing an important role in the diagnosis of arterial stenosis of the lower limbs, with sensitivity and specificity rates of around 95% **[48]**. Compared with arteriography, which remains the reference examination, it has the advantage of not involving the injection of nephrotoxic iodinated contrast products. It provides sufficient information to guide treatment. Recently, there have been reports **[49] of cases of** "nephrogenic systemic fibrosis" secondary to the administration of gadolinium chelates, particularly gadodiamide, in patients with acute or chronic renal failure. Therefore, if gadolinium is to be administered to a diabetic patient with renal insufficiency, a product other than gadodiamide should be used, at the lowest possible dose and with any dialysis sessions after gadolinium administration intensified.

2.1.3.3. Arteriography

Intra-arterial angiography provides images of excellent quality, enabling endovascular revascularisation procedures to be carried out afterwards. However, it is invasive, costly and carries the risk of complications (5% compared with 0.5% for MRI angiography), in particular renal failure induced by iodinated contrast products. It requires prior assessment of renal function and glycaemic control, stopping diuretics and hydrating the patient 12 hours before and after the examination. It is the imaging of last resort when non-invasive imaging (MRI or even angioscan) has not provided all the information required to plan a possible surgical bypass; it is essential when endovascular revascularisation is envisaged.

3. Infection

Infection is the aggravating factor in diabetic ulcers; it can progress rapidly and constitute an emergency. Clinical examination of the feet should systematically look for an entry point (ulcer, periungual or interdigital lesion). Any general signs should be noted: temperature, increased heart rate and respiratory rate. Biological examinations will analyse diabetes control, blood count, sedimentation rate and CRP (C-reactive protein) levels.

3.1. Clinical examination

Redness, swelling and erythema indicate soft tissue inflammation. The infection is often deeper than first thought. An erythematous, oedematous "sausage-like" appearance of a toe is also suggestive of osteoarthritis. All ulcers should be examined with a sterile stylet or forceps: if there is a "rough" bone contact, this is evidence of osteitis or osteoarthritis until proven otherwise.

3.2. Bacteriological analysis

When there are no clinical signs of infection, it is not recommended to take bacteriological samples, the culture of which would only reveal a "normal" infection. However, in the presence of a superficial or deep infection, a bacteriological examination is essential. The difficulty in managing infected diabetic foot wounds lies in the need to differentiate between infection and colonisation, and therefore to know when and how to take a microbiological sample[16]. The aim of bacteriological analysis is to identify the bacteria responsible for the infection and to study their sensitivity to antibiotics.

3.2.1. Withdrawals

Bacteriological sampling is only indicated in the case of clinically established infection. Wounds without clinical signs (local or general) of infection (IWGDF grade 1) should not be sampled. Multidisciplinary management of these patients is essential. Sampling protocols must be devised jointly by clinicians, surgeons and microbiologists in accordance with the recommendations below (Table 7). There is no consensus on the best sampling technique to use, due to a lack of sufficient studies. Samples should not be inoculated into blood culture bottles due to the presence of non-pathogenic commensal flora[16, 17].

Table 7. Recommendations for microbiological sampling of foot wounds in diabetics[17].

To do
Bacteriological samples should only be taken if the wound infection is clinically confirmed (PEDIS grade 2-4). Clean and debride the wound (surgically or mechanically) before taking any samplesObtain a tissue sample, either by scraping with a sterile scalpel or curette, or by using a biopsy punch at the base of the debrided wound. Aspirate purulent secretions using a syringe and a sterile needle, passing through healthy skin.
For suspected osteitis, perform a bone biopsy, either in the operating theatre, or by percutaneous ultrasound or radioguided sampling through the healthy skin. Promptly transfer the samples to a sterile jar with a few drops of sterile serum (to avoid drying out) or to a suitable transport medium, for aerobic/anaerobic cultures (and Gram staining if possible). Repeat sampling only if the infection does not clear up despite antibiotics or if the infection is severe
What not to do
Remove a colonised wound (PEDIS grade 1) Obtain a sample without cleaning or debridement of the wound Take a sample by simple swabbing Take a superficial swab when the infection is deep-rooted

3.2.1.1. Production

3.2.1.1.1. Debridement

Lesions are always superficially colonised by bacterial flora which do not necessarily have pathological significance. This is why the wound must be prepared before any sampling. The aim of debridement is to excise necrotic soft tissue, devitalised and contaminated tissue and fibrous tissue, leaving only healthy tissue in place to facilitate wound healing (tissue re-epithelialisation is encouraged).

The extent of debridement will depend on the type of ulceration:

- Ulcerations that are predominantly neuropathic: debridement must be continued until the healthy tissue is reached, and this can be done easily due to the absence of pain;
- Ischaemic ulcers: debridement must be very cautious and limited to simple drainage. It is recommended that vascular management be carried out before any bacteriological investigation.

Two types of samples can be taken:
- Surgical: this is the most effective sampling in terms of microbiological documentation. It must be taken in the operating theatre by a

specialist surgeon under rigorous aseptic conditions. This debridement has diagnostic (exploration of the various compartments of the foot to see how far the infection has spread), prognostic (taking reliable bacteriological samples), therapeutic (removal of necrotic tissue and reduction of bacterial inoculum) and preventive (correction of foot deformities to avoid recurrence) aims;
- Mechanical: the sample is taken in the patient's bed by a doctor or specialist nurse, using a sterile scalpel or curette. The area is cleaned with sterile saline gauze. Antiseptics may be used; they should be applied to the edges of the wound and then removed with sterile saline before the sample is taken. They help to limit/eliminate the skin commensal microflora[16 17].

3.2.1.1.2. Specimens in cases of soft tissue infection

Sampling methods are adapted to the nature of the lesions. From the outset, it should be noted that superficial swabbing of the wound is the least effective sampling technique.

- Superficial wounds

In these cases, a superficial swab of the wound is taken at the patient's bedside. This is the most commonly used sampling method, but it is not very reliable. It is poorly suited to identifying the bacteria actually responsible for the infection. No methodology has been validated. Most commonly, a swab is passed over a 1 cm^2 area of the wound in a zigzag movement combined with a rotating motion. This method collects bacteria, but it is then difficult to distinguish the flora from the bacteria. colonisation of the bacteria responsible for the infection. This is why it should only be performed in Grade 2 infections, under very strict conditions to avoid contamination: careful debridement of necrotic tissue, washing of the foot with water and mild soap, then rinsing of the wound with physiological saline. In all cases, the swab must be placed in a transport medium.This type of sample is not tested for strict anaerobic bacteria. It must be repeated several times during the consultation. In order for the samples to be relevant, several concordant results must be available.

- **Deep wounds**

o **Tissue biopsy**

This is the preferred method. It can be performed in the patient's bed, especially in cases of severe neuropathy, after preparing the skin (debridement, excision of necrotic tissue after careful cleaning). Two to four fragments of tissue are removed (using a "punch biopsy" to obtain a tissue core) from different areas depending on the extent of the wound, and placed immediately in a sterile jar (with a few drops of sterile saline added to prevent drying out) or a transport medium (if the laboratory is at a distance). This type of sample must be tested for strict anaerobic bacteria.

o **Aspiration with a fine needle or long catheter**

This procedure allows deep wounds to be punctured, particularly in the case of collected infections. The puncture is made through a previously disinfected healthy area (either percutaneously or under ultrasound control). If no liquid is aspirated, 1 to 2 ml of physiological serum is injected and aspirated using a second needle. In all cases, the syringe (of the type used to measure blood gases) used for sampling is quickly sent to the laboratory without the needle, purged of air and hermetically and sterile sealed. This type of sample must be tested for strict anaerobic bacteria.

o **Curettage - deep swabbing of the ulcer**

Tissue is removed by scraping the base of the ulcer with a sterile curette. The curettage products are recovered by swabbing. The swab is immediately placed in a transport medium and sent rapidly to the laboratory. This type of sample is not tested for strict anaerobic bacteria.

3.2.1.1.3. Samples to be taken in cases of acute osteitis

They are carried out by bone biopsy, which is the reference method. It is quick, simple and has no side effects, but must be carried out in specialist centres by specialist doctors/surgeons. The biopsy should be carried out after a therapeutic window of at least 15 days if antibiotic therapy has been started beforehand.
A bone biopsy can be obtained :

- By surgery (reference method) in the operating theatre if the centre has a surgeon specialising in this procedure. A maximum of five samples should be taken from the lesion;
- Percutaneous radio-, ultrasound-guided or CT-guided puncture performed by a radiologist by passing the trocar (of the myelogram type) through the healthy skin after disinfecting it as thoroughly as possible. This procedure can be carried out without a local anaesthetic in many diabetic patients because of their sensory neuropathy. Several areas can be sampled. The sample must be placed in a sterile jar or transport medium (if the laboratory is at a distance).

Whatever the technique used, the sample must be suitable for aerobic and anaerobic culture. For aerobic culture, a small amount of sterile saline is added to the sample to prevent drying. A transport medium can also be used for aerobic culture. A histopathological examination may complete the analysis. This should be interpreted by a pathologist specialising in this field **[16, 17]**.

3.2.1.1.4. Aerobic and anaerobic blood cultures

They are performed in cases of severe sepsis (IWGDF grade 4).

3.2.1.1.5. Transport

This requires close collaboration between clinicians, nurses and couriers, because of the significant risk of desiccation and bacterial lysis. The transport medium is especially necessary when testing for anaerobic bacteria (deep sampling) on small-volume biopsies (< 1 cm).[2]

3.2.1.1.6. Interpretation

Interpreting the results is rarely straightforward. It depends on the nature of the sample and the quality of the sampling, packaging and transport. It also depends on the nature of the bacteria isolated. All of these factors need to be taken into account if the bacteria detected are to be incriminated in the infection (Table 8).

Table 8. Clinical-bacteriological correlation between wound types and bacteria involved and identified [17].

Type of foot wound	Pathogens
Recent superficial wound without antibiotic therapy recent	Staphylococcus aureus β-hemolytic Streptococci
Chronic wound (≥ 1 month) or previously treated with antibiotics	Staphylococcus aureus β-hemolytic Streptococci
	Enterobacteriaceae
Wound treated with evolving cephalosporins unfavourable	Enterococci
Macerated lesion	Pseudomonasspp. (in association with other micro-organisms)
Long-term wound (ulcer ≥ 6 months), previous treatment with broad-spectrum antibiotics	Polymicrobism: aerobic Gram-positive cocci (Staphylococcus aureus, β-haemolytic streptococci,SCN, enterococci), corynebacteria, enterobacteria, Pseudomonasspp. and Gram-negative bacilli that are not aerobic. fermentative +/- fungal agents
Nauseating odour, necrosis, gangrene	Gram-positive aerobic cocci, enterobacteria, Pseudomonasspp., non-fermentative Gram-negative bacilli, strict anaerobes

SC: coagulase-negative staphylococci.

In the first instance, commensal or colonising bacteria are not taken into account. These include coagulase-negative staphylococci, corynebacteria, enterococci and Pseudomonas aeruginosa. Their pathogenic role must always be discussed, especially in the case of superficial infections. However, these bacteria can also act as opportunistic pathogens (particularly when detected in deep bone samples; Table 8). There are no criteria for being certain that the bacteria isolated are responsible for the clinically observed infection. However, bacteria of low virulence or commensal bacteria are taken into account if they are isolated on several occasions, from repeated high-quality samples, or if the patient presents a worrying septic state. Gram-positive bacteria are the most common pathogens. These are often Staphylococcus aureus in pure or poly-microbial culture, in superficial or deep wounds. Beta haemolytic streptococci are frequently isolated, often in association with other bacteria. Gram-negative bacilli isolated in this context are most often enterobacteria (Proteus mirabilis, Escherichia coli, Klebsiellaspp.) which are observed in deep, chronic or previously treated infections. Strict anaerobic bacteria are very diverse and often associated with facultative aerobic-anaerobic bacteria. Finegoldia magna and Bacteroidesspp. are the most pathogenic. Metagenomic studies of wounds show that these bacteria are constantly present in deep wounds. An antibiotic susceptibility test should be carried out on bacteria considered to be pathogenic (Table 9). The bacteria isolated may be multi-resistant, especially when the patient has been hospitalised several times. Isolation of methicillin-resistant S. aureus (MRSA) is not synonymous with increased virulence[16]. In conclusion, diabetic foot wound infections are the main cause of hospitalisation for diabetics and one of the major causes of lower-limb amputations. This condition is a real public health problem, and rapid diagnosis and effective treatment are essential. The identification and management of foot wound infections in diabetics are often problematic due to difficulties in :

- Differentiation between infection and colonisation ;

- Assessment of the extent of the infection ;

- The implementation of an effective treatment due to the increase in the frequency of multi-resistant bacteria and the alteration in the pharmacokinetic properties of antibiotics due to the poor vascular condition of the arteries in the patient's foot;

- The duration of treatment, as this has not been clearly defined due to a lack of studies (particularly in the case of osteitis).

However, the development of clinical criteria to recognise and classify the severity of foot wound infections in diabetics, the optimisation of sampling techniques by favouring deep samples, the development of rapid molecular biology techniques to analyse the The virulence and resistance potential of pathogens and the availability of new anti-S. aureus antibiotics may help clinicians in the future to improve the management of these pathogens[17].

Table 9. Bacteria involved in superficial and deep infections of the diabetic foot for which an antibiogram can be performed [16].

Gram-positive bacteria (the more frequent)	S. aureus, streptococcus beta haemolytic	Antibiogram to be performed
	Enterococci	Antibiogram to be discussed in depending on the pathogenic role and the quality of the sample
Gram-negative bacteria	Enterobacteriaceae (mainly) :P. mirabilis, E. coli, Klebsiellaspp.	Antibiogram to be performed
	P. aeruginosa	Antibiogram to be discussed in depending on the pathogenic role and the quality of the sample
Anaerobes	Gram positive (most often) Gram negative (Bacteroidesetc)	Antibiogram to be carried out systematically in cases of antimicrobial infection or according to the species isolated during polymicrobial infection

3.3. Osteoarticular imaging

Infection can be assessed using standard X-rays, ultrasound, CT scans, magnetic resonance imaging (MRI) and isotope examinations.

3.3.1. Standard radiography

Signs of osteitis are delayed in relation to the onset of infection, and it is sometimes difficult to distinguish osteitis lesions from neuroarthropathy lesions (Charcot's foot). However, the metaphysiodiaphyseal lytic appearance is relatively typical of osteitis, especially in the of the forefoot. It is recommended that standard X-rays be taken systematically in the case of ulcers, and re-evaluated comparatively 8 to 15 days later in the case of suspected osteitis: in the case of osteitis, osteolysis that is initially absent will be visible 15 days later. This is a simple, inexpensive, reproducible comparative examination which is essential in the evaluation of osteoarticular infections. In a study **[50] of** the diagnosis of osteitis confirmed by histology of bone samples taken during the operation, plain radiographs performed well (accurate diagnosis 79%, sensitivity 87%, false negatives 12%). This was also the case for bone scintigraphy using labelled polynuclear cells (accurate diagnosis 93%, sensitivity 93%, false negatives 7%), although it did not really provide any additional information compared with plain radiographs.

3.3.2. Scanner

It is useful for confirming osteolysis when radiography is doubtful. This is particularly the case in the midfoot or hindfoot.

3.3.3. MRI with gadolinium injection

The literature [51] recognises it as a good test for diagnosing osteitis. It can be used to differentiate osteoarthritic lesions from those of neurogenic osteoarthropathy [52]. It is a very sensitive test, but its specificity is much less good. Similarly, it is reserved for "acute" feet. "with cellulitis. It is the examination of choice for diagnosing deep collections of soft tissue and their diffusion into tendon sheaths, and can be used to guide surgical drainage.

3.3.4. Ultrasound

It is easier to access and less expensive. It can also be used to diagnose collections or abscesses, and to guide puncture for bacteriological purposes.

3.3.5. Isotopic examinations

In the event of diagnostic doubt on plain radiographs and/or CT scan, technetium bone scintigraphy coupled with labelled polynuclear cells is the test of choice for diagnosing osteitis. Combining the two methods would give a sensitivity close to 100% and a specificity greater than 95% [53]. In the coming years, the diagnostic potential of PET-scan will be further developed; in particular, it is better at locating the site of infection than standard scintigraphic examinations.

VI.CARE

According to the recommendations of the International Consensus on the Diabetic Foot published in 1999 by the IWGDF (updated 2019), prevention and treatment of diabetic foot complications should be organised on three levels. In all countries, there should be at least three levels of diabetic foot management with a multidisciplinary group of specialists.

Level 1: GPs, diabetes nurses and chiropodistsThe aim is to make diabetics aware of foot problems and how to prevent them, and to diagnose ulcers at an early stage.

Level 2: diabetologists, diabetes nurses, surgeons (general and/or vascular and/or orthopaedic), surgeons (general, orthopaedic or foot specialists), vascular specialists (endovascular and open revascularisation), infectious disease specialists or clinical microbiologists, podiatrists and diabetes nurses, in collaboration with a shoemaker, orthotist or prosthetist.It covers basic preventive and curative care for the diabetic foot. General practitioners should be able to refer their patients to these centres. Depending on their skills and the diagnostic resources available to them, they should be able to refer the most difficult cases to the centres of reference.

Level 3: Reference centres: A level 2 foot centre specialising in diabetic foot care, with multiple experts from several disciplines each specialising in this field working together, and which acts as a tertiary reference centre.These centres should have close multidisciplinary collaboration between diabetologists, orthopaedic surgeons and vascular surgeons. They deal with the most difficult cases: deep, infected ulcers, severe arteriopathy, Charcot's foot.Studies conducted throughout the world have shown that setting up a multidisciplinary foot care team and implementing prevention and management of diabetic foot disease is associated with a reduction in the frequency of diabetes-related lower limb amputations. If it is not possible to create a complete team from the outset, we should try to build one step by step and introduce the various possible disciplines. Above all, this team should act with mutual respect and work in both primary and secondary care settings, with at least one member available for consultation or patient assessment at all times.Faced with the growing incidence of diabetes and the resulting economic costs, the various countries must prepare to manage this pandemic. The reality is often far from this ideal: in 2008, the results of the prospective European study **[54]** carried out in 14 centres still showed treatments that did not comply with international recommendations, and the persistence of major variations between countries and centres. Several studies have shown that less than 50% of diabetics have had an annual foot examination, either by their general practitioner or by their diabetologist [55, 56], and that foot checks at home are still inadequate, ranging from 20 to 70%.Belgium has been at the forefront of the organisation of diabetic foot care, with the creation in 1989 of the first two university centres for diabetic foot care. multidisciplinary care of the diabetic foot. At present, the diabetic passport provides level 1 care, including in particular chiropody. The diabetes convention centres meet the criteria for level 2 and, above all, Belgium has 22 multidisciplinary diabetic foot centres approved in 2005, providing a structured range of care [57, 58].The management of diabetic feet is costly in terms of highly specialised staff and care. This condition is very poorly valued. Yet the role of the public authorities should be decisive in encouraging the development of centres of reference. This lack of interest is characterised by the fact that no reliable statistics, either medical or economic, are available on the importance of the diabetic foot in Algeria.Prevention is the only way to reduce the incidence of ulcers, amputations and the cost of diabetic feet.The treatment of diabetic feet is usually a multidisciplinary process involving different specialities. The vascular and infectious assessment of diabetic ulcers enables a suitable treatment to be proposed.IWGDF 2019 describes the basic principles of diabetic foot ulcer prevention and management based on:

-Prevention of foot ulcers in people with diabetes [59] ;

-Discharge of foot ulcers in people with diabetes [60] ;

-Diagnosis, prognosis and management of peripheral arterial disease in patients with foot ulcers and diabetes [61] ;

- Diagnosis and treatment of foot infections in people with diabetes [62] ;

-Surgical interventions to improve healing of foot ulcers in people with diabetes [63] ;

-Classification of diabetic foot ulcers [64].

1.Preventing foot ulcers

Efforts to prevent foot ulcers are based on five key elements:

-Identifying the foot at risk ;

-Inspect and examine the foot at risk regularly;

-Educating patients, families and healthcare professionals;

-Ensure that appropriate footwear is worn regularly;

-Treat risk factors for ulceration.

A team of trained healthcare professionals should address these five elements as part of integrated care for people at high risk of ulceration (IWGDF 3 risk).

1.1.Identifying the foot at risk

The absence of symptoms in a person with diabetes does not rule out a foot ulcer; they may have asymptomatic neuropathy, arteriopathy, pre-ulcer signs or even an ulcer. Examine a person with diabetes at very low risk of foot ulceration (IWGDF 0 risk) annually for signs or symptoms of loss of protective sensation and arteriopathy, to identify whether they are at risk of ulceration and look for the following:
-Past history: ulcer / amputation of lower limbs, claudication;

-Vascular status: palpation of pedal and posterior tibial pulses;

- Loss of protective sensitivity: assess with one of the following techniques:

✓ Pressure perception: monofilamentWomen-Weinstein 10 grams ;

✓ Vibration perception: 128 Hz tuning fork;

✓ When the monofilament or tuning fork is not available, test tactile sensation: lightly touch the tip of the patient's toes with the tip of your index finger for 1 to 2 seconds.

1.2. Regular inspection and examination of the foot at risk (IWGDF 1 or higher)

In a diabetic patient with loss of protective sensitivity or arterial disease (IWGDF risk 1-3), carry out a more complete examination, including the following:

- History of: lower limb ulcer/amputation, end-stage renal disease, previous foot education, social isolation, poor access to healthcare and financial constraints, painful foot (when walking or resting) or numbness, claudication;
-Vascular status: palpation of pedal pulses;

-Skin: assessment of skin colour, temperature, presence of calluses or oedema, pre-ulcer signs;
-Bones/joints: look for deformities (e.g. claw or hammer toes), abnormally large bony prominences, or limited joint mobility. Examine the patient's feet both lying down and standing up;

- Assessment of the loss of protective sensitivity, if sensitivity was intact during a previous examination;

-Shoes: ill-fitting, inadequate or insufficient;

- Poor foot hygiene, e.g. badly cut nails, unwashed feet, superficial fungal infection or dirty socks;

- Physical limitations that may affect personal foot care (e.g. visual acuity, obesity);

-Knowledge of foot care.

Following examination of the foot, classify each patient using the IWGDF risk classification system shown in Table 10 to guide the frequency and management of subsequent preventive screening. The areas of the foot most at risk are illustrated in Figure 3. Any foot ulcers identified during screening should be treated according to the principles set out below.

Table 10. The 2019 IWGDF risk classification system and corresponding foot screening frequency[39].

Category	Risk of ulcers	Features	Frequency *
0	Very low	No neuropathy and no arterial disease	Once a year
1	Low	Neuropathy or low arteriopathy	Once every 6-12 month
2	Moderate	Neuropathy moderate + arterial disease Or Neuropathy + foot deformity Or Arterial disease + foot deformity	Once every 3-6 months
3	Severe	Neuropathy or arterial disease and one or more of the following: History of foot Lower limb amputation (minor or major) Terminal phase of kidney disease	Once every 1 to 3 months

*The frequency of screening is based on expert opinion, as there is no published evidence to support these intervals.

1.3. Informing patients, families and healthcare professionals about foot care

Education, presented in a structured, organised and repeated manner, is widely considered to play an important role in the prevention of diabetic foot ulcers. The aim is to improve the patient's self-care of the foot, self-protection knowledge and behaviour, and to improve their motivation and skills to facilitate adherence to this behaviour. People with diabetes, particularly those at risk of IWGDF 1 or more, need to learn how to recognise foot ulcers and how to treat them. The educator should demonstrate patient-specific skills, such as how to cut toenails correctly. The educator should demonstrate patient-specific skills, such as how to cut toenails correctly (Figure 13).A member of the healthcare team should provide structured education (see sample instructions below) individually or in small groups in multiple sessions, with periodic reinforcement, and preferably using a mixture of methods. Structured education should be culturally appropriate, taking into account gender differences. It is essential to assess whether the person with diabetes (and, optimally, any close family members or carers) has understood the messages, is motivated to act and adhere to the advice, to ensure sufficient self-care skills. In addition, healthcare professionals providing these instructions should receive periodic training to improve their own skills in caring for people at high risk of foot ulceration.

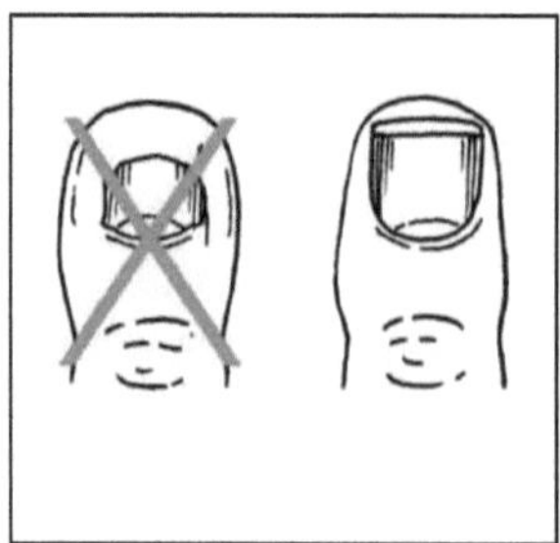

Figure 13. The correct way to cut toenails [39].

The elements to be covered when educating the person at risk of foot ulceration (IWGDF risk 1 or more) are:

-Determine whether the person is able to inspect their feet. If not, discuss with people who can help with this task. Visit people who have a significant visual impairment or a physical inability to see their feet cannot do the inspection properly;

-Explain the need for a daily foot inspection of the entire surface of both feet, including the areas between the toes;

- Ensure that the patient knows how to notify the appropriate healthcare professional if the measured foot temperature is significantly increased, or if a blister, cut, scrape or ulcer has developed;

-Review the following practices with the patient:

✓ Avoid walking barefoot, in socks without shoes, or in thin-soled slippers, whether at home or out and about;

✓ Do not wear shoes that are too tight, have rough edges or uneven seams;

✓ Visually inspect and manually feel the inside of all shoes before putting them on;

✓ Wear socks without seams (or with the seams inside out); do not wear tight or knee-high socks) and change your socks every day;

✓ Wash your feet every day (with the water temperature always below 37°C) and dry them thoroughly, especially between the toes;

✓ Do not use heaters or hot water bottles to warm your feet;

✓ Do not use chemical agents or plasters to eliminate corns and calluses; see the appropriate health professional for these problems;

✓ Use emollients to lubricate dry skin, but not between the toes;

✓ Cut the toenails straight across (Figure 13);

✓ Have your feet examined regularly by a health professional

1.4. Ensuring that appropriate footwear is worn regularly

In people with diabetes and insensitive feet, wearing inappropriate footwear or walking barefoot are the main causes of foot trauma leading to foot ulceration. The person who has lost protective sensitivity must have and should be encouraged to wear appropriate footwear at all times, both indoors and outdoors (and may need financial assistance to acquire it). All footwear must be suitable and conform to any changes in foot structure or foot biomechanics affecting the person's foot. The person with protective sensitivity or without arteriopathy (IWGDF 0) can select well-fitting off-the-shelf shoes. People with protective sensitivity or neuropathy (IWGDF 1-3) must take great care when selecting or fitting shoes; this is particularly important when they also have foot deformities (IWGDF 2) or a history of ulcers/amputations (IWGDF 3).

The inside length of the shoe should be 1 to 2 cm longer than the foot, and should not be too tight or too loose (Figure 14). The internal width should be equal to the width of the foot at the metatarsophalangeal joints (or the widest part of the foot), and the height should leave enough room for all the toes. Assess the fit with the patient in a standing position, preferably later in the day (when they can with swollen feet). If there are no off-the-shelf shoes that can accommodate the foot (for example, if the fit is poor due to foot deformity) or if there are signs of abnormal foot loading (for example, hyperaemia, calluses, ulceration), refer the patient to special shoe fitters (advice and/or construction), possibly including extra-deep shoes, custom-made shoes, insoles or orthoses.

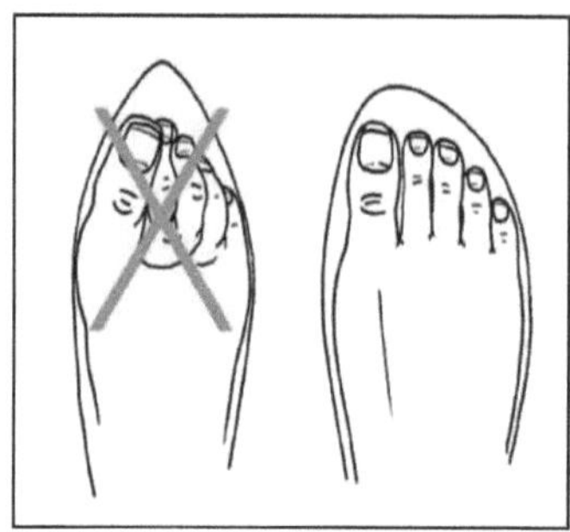

Figure 14. Shoes should be wide enough to accommodate the foot without excessive pressure on the skin [39].

To prevent a recurrent plantar foot ulcer, ensure that the patient's therapeutic footwear has been shown to relieve plantar pressure during walking. Ask the patient never to wear the same shoe that caused the ulcer in the first place.

1.5. Treatment of risk factors for ulceration

In a diabetic patient, treat any modifiable risk factors or pre-ulcer signs in the foot. This includes: removing excessive calluses; protecting blisters or emptying them if necessary; treating ingrown or thickened toenails appropriately; and prescribing antifungal treatment for fungal infections. This treatment should be repeated until these abnormalities disappear and do not recur over time, and carried out by a suitably trained healthcare professional. In patients with recurrent ulcers due to foot deformities that develop despite the optimal preventive measures described above, surgical intervention should be considered.

2.Principles of ulcer treatment

Treatment involves offloading the affected foot, cleaning the wound and detersion (debridement), then covering the wound.

2.1.Foot release

This is the essential and fundamental therapeutic measure, without which healing becomes illusory. The use of expensive dressings or even new biotechnological approaches (growth factors, living skin substitutes, etc.) is useless if the two basic principles, removal of local pressure and debridement of the wound, are not respected.

2.1.1.Discharge boots

Total contact cast. This is the reference treatment for ulcers and the acute phase of Charcot foot. Its aim is to distribute pressure evenly over the arch of the foot during all phases of walking; 30 to 50% of pressure is absorbed by the cast [65]. The fact that it cannot be removed 24 hours a day is an essential factor in its success, and allows healing to be achieved in 70 to 85% of cases. However, it must be made up by highly experienced personnel according to a highly codified procedure: interdigital protection for each toe, protective foam for the malleoli and tibial crest, plaster that is easier to mould than synthetic resins (to be used only as a covering and reinforcing layer), and a walking heel pad. Its effectiveness in reducing plantar pressure and healing is better in the forefoot and midfoot than in the hindfoot [66], although devices such as rubber rocker heels added under the plaster have been proposed to compensate for the lack of relief from full-contact plaster for hindfoot ulcers [67]. It must be changed every week. The rate of complications varies from 5 to 30% [68]: friction lesions that can lead to new infected wounds, interdigital mycotic infections, venous thrombosis, etc.

2.1.2.Other landfill systems

The effectiveness in terms of offloading of the different devices is not equivalent [69], including between the different commercially available removable boots [70]. Because of compliance problems, non-removable boots are thought to provide shorter healing times than offloading shoes or pneumatic boots [71]. However, even if the total contact cast remains the gold standard in the IWGDF consensus, it is only used by a few specialist teams: a study in 2005 [72] showed that it was used by less than 2% of 895 centres (50 states in the United States) treating diabetic feet. At the Saint-Luc University Centre in Brussels, total contact plaster is the treatment of choice for acute Charcot ulcers and feet [57, 58].

2.2. Restoring tissue perfusion

Before considering treatment of a diabetic ulcer, it is essential to correct vascular insufficiency. No indication for amputation or orthopaedic surgery should be given without a precise assessment of the vascular condition of the patient's lower limbs. Critical ischaemia of the lower limbs in diabetics is clinically manifested by an ulcer with an element of necrosis, decubitus pain or intermittent claudication, but is less frequent than in non-diabetics because of the associated neuropathy. Revascularisation, where possible, remains the key to ulcer healing, as it allows tissue oxygenation and better diffusion of antibiotics.

In practice, in the presence of an ulcer, the vascular assessment should include a Doppler and, if possible, a measurement of TcPO2; if it is less than 30 mm Hg, a vascular opinion is essential (P3 in the PEDIS classification). Depending on the results of additional tests (angio-MRI or arteriography), the possibility of revascularisation may be discussed (Figure 15). Critical ischaemia is an indication for revascularisation, either surgically or using endovascular techniques. Hyperbaric oxygen therapy may be recommended for ulcers associated with severe non-revascularisable arteritis.

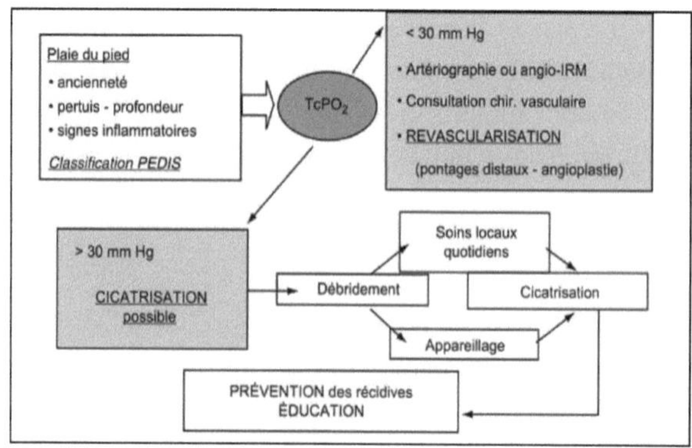

Figure 15. The role of vascular surgery

2.3. Treatment of the infection

-Superficial ulcer with limited soft tissue infection (mild):

✓ Clean and debride all necrotic tissue and calluses;

✓ Start empirical oral antibiotic therapy targeting Staphylococcus aureus and streptococci).

-Deep or extensive (potentially limb-threatening) infection (moderate or severe infection):

✓ Urgently assess the need for surgery to remove necrotic tissue, including infected bone, remove compartment pressure or drain abscesses;

✓ Initiate empirical, parenteral, broad-spectrum antibiotic therapy for Gram-positive and Gram-negative bacteria, including strict anaerobic bacteria;

✓ Adjust the antibiotic regimen according to both the clinical response to empirical therapy and the culture and sensitivity results.

2.4. Metabolic control and treatment of co-morbidities

-Optimise blood sugar control, if necessary with insulin;

-Treat any oedema or malnutrition.

2.5. Local ulcer care

2.5.1. Wound cleansing and detersion

When caring for diabetic feet, it is important to stress the importance of good general hygiene, and in particular daily foot washing, followed by careful drying. Care of the wound begins with disinfection of the wound and surrounding area with a careful wash in water, followed by treatment with antiseptics; polyiodinated solutions are more effective than chlorhexidine and do not alter healing, while avoiding the risk of the emergence of resistant germs [MRSA (methicillin-resistant Staphylococcus aureus and others)][58]. The administration of local antibiotics should be avoided for the same reasons. All ulcers require limited debridement, which consists of mechanically removing the callus around the ulcer with a scalpel blade. Once the edges have been debrided, the wound can be delineated with a curette to remove necrotic, yellowish residues and fibrin. This mechanical detersion is essential to encourage budding. Some ulcers may require necrotic structures to be removed and trimmed surgically. Dressings also help to detoxify devitalised tissue.

2.6. Place of surgery

In the context of these D1 and D2 lesions in the PEDIS classification, orthopaedic surgery may be indicated to facilitate the healing of intractable forefoot ulcers or prevent their recurrence. Percutaneous lengthening of the Achilles tendon or sectioning of the gastrocnemius fascia (Strayer procedure) may be considered and discussed in cases of ankle stiffness with absence of dorsiflexion or even slight equinus [73, 74]. Similarly, metatarsal elevation osteotomies (particularly of the first radius) in cases of hyper-support maintained by a static disorder or distal percutaneous osteotomies of the lateral metatarsals are possible to reduce hyper-support in relation to an ulcer. The aim of these procedures is to reduce mechanical stress on the forefoot. In the case of significant loss of substance after trimming, plastic surgery is also an option, provided that the vascular condition is satisfactory (P1, P2 in the PEDIS classification) and that it is possible to modify the hyperpressure factors. This may involve a small bilobed rotational flap after resection of a plantar ulceration, or local sural-type flaps, among others, for the after-effects of heel pressure sores.

2.7. Patient and family education

- Educate patients (and their relatives or carers) about appropriate personal care for foot ulcers and how to recognise and report signs and symptoms of new infection or signs of worsening (e.g. onset of fever, wound condition, worsening hyperglycaemia).
- During a period of enforced bed rest (complete bed rest), explain how to prevent another foot ulcer.

3. Assessment and classification of foot ulcers

Healthcare professionals should follow a standardised and consistent strategy when assessing a foot ulcer, as this will guide further assessment and therapy. The following points should be addressed:

3.1. Type

On the basis of the history and clinical examination, classify the ulcer as neuropathic, neuro-ischaemic or ischaemic. Loss of sensation is characteristic of a neuropathic ulcer. Also look for the presence of arteriopathy and palpate the pedal pulses. That said, there are no specific symptoms or signs of arteriopathy that reliably indicate healing of the ulcer. Therefore, examine the waveforms of the pedal artery and measure the ankle-brachial index (ABI) using a Doppler instrument. The presence of an ABI of 0.9-1.3 or a triphasic pedal pulse waveform largely excludes arteriopathy.

3.2. Cause

Wearing ill-fitting shoes and walking barefoot are practices that frequently lead to foot ulceration, even in patients with exclusively ischaemic ulcers. It is therefore essential to carefully examine the footwear and behaviour of every patient suffering from a foot ulcer.

3.3. Site and depth

Neuropathic ulcers most commonly develop on the plantar surface of the foot, or in areas overlying a bony deformity. Ischaemic and neuro-ischaemic ulcers develop more frequently on the tips of the toes or the lateral edges of the foot.
Determining the depth of a foot ulcer can be difficult, particularly in the presence of overlying callus or necrotic tissue. To facilitate assessment of the ulcer, any neuropathic or neuro-ischaemic ulcer surrounded by callus or containing necrotic soft tissue should be debrided at initial presentation or as soon as possible. However, do not debride a non-infected ulcer that shows signs of severe ischaemia. Neuropathic ulcers can usually be debrided without the need for local anaesthetic.

3.4. Signs of infection

Foot infection in a person with diabetes poses a serious threat to the affected foot and limb and must be assessed and treated promptly. Because all ulcers are colonised by potential pathogens, infection is diagnosed by the presence of at least two signs or symptoms of inflammation (redness, warmth, induration, pain/tenderness) or purulent secretions. Unfortunately, these signs may be attenuated by neuropathy or ischaemia, and systemic signs (e.g. pain, fever, leucocytosis) are often absent and the infection moderate. Infections should be classified according to the IDSA / IWGDF scheme as mild (superficial with minimal cellulitis), moderate (deeper or more extensive) or severe (accompanied by systemic signs of sepsis), as well as whether or not they are accompanied by osteitis [62]. If not properly treated, the infection can spread contiguously to underlying tissues, including bone (osteitis). Assess patients with diabetic foot infection for the presence of osteomyelitis, particularly if the ulcer is old, deep or located directly on a prominent bone. Examine the ulcer to determine whether it is possible to visualise or touch the bone with a sterile metal probe. In addition to clinical assessment, consider obtaining plain radiographs in most patients to look for evidence of osteomyelitis, tissue gas or foreign body. Where more advanced imaging is required, consider MRI, or for those in whom this is not possible, other techniques (e.g. radionuclides or PET scan).For clinically infected wounds, obtain a tissue sample for culture (and a Gram-stained smear, if available); avoid obtaining samples for wound cultures with a swab. The pathogens responsible for foot infection (and their susceptibilities to antibiotics) vary according to geographical, demographic and social situations. Staphylococcus aureus (alone or in association with other microorganisms) is the predominant pathogen in most cases. Chronic and more severe infections are often polymicrobial, with aerobic Gram-negative and anaerobic bacilli accompanying Gram-positive cocci, particularly in warmer climates.

3.5. Patient factors

In addition to a systematic assessment of the ulcer, foot and leg, patient-related factors that may affect wound healing, such as end-stage renal disease, oedema, malnutrition, metabolic control or psychosocial problems, must also be taken into account.

3.6. Classification of ulcers

Assess the severity of infection using the IWGDF/ISDA classification criteria [62, 64] and in patients with neuropathy, it is recommended that the WIfI (wound/ischaemia/infection) system be used to classify the risk of amputation and the benefit of revascularisation [61, 64].For communication between healthcare professionals, the SINBAD System is recommended, which can also be used for auditing population outcomes [64].

4. Organisation of diabetic foot care

Successful efforts to prevent and treat diabetic foot disease depend on a well-organised team, using a holistic approach in which the ulcer is seen as a sign of multi-organ disease, and integrating the different disciplines involved. Effective organisation requires systems and guidelines for education, screening, risk reduction, treatment and audit. Local variations in resources and staffing often dictate how care is delivered, but Ideally, a diabetic foot disease programme should provide the following elements:

- Education for people with diabetes and their carers, hospital health staff and healthcare professionals;

-Systems to detect all those at risk, including an annual foot examination for all diabetics;

-Access to measures to reduce the risk of foot ulceration, such as podiatric care and the provision of appropriate footwear;

-Quick access to fast, effective treatment for any foot ulcer or infection;

-Audit all aspects of the service to identify and resolve problems and ensure that local practices meet accepted standards of care;

- A comprehensive structure designed to meet the needs of patients requiring chronic care, rather than simply responding to acute problems as they arise.

In all countries, there should be at least three levels of foot care management with multidisciplinary specialists such as those listed in Table 11.

Table 11. Levels of care for diabetic foot disease [39].

Level of care	Interdisciplinary specialists involved
Level 1	General practitioner, podiatrist and nurse in diabetology
Level 2	Diabetologist, surgeon (general, orthopaedic or foot), vascular specialist (endovascular and open revascularisation), infectious disease specialist or clinical microbiologist, podiatrist and diabetes nurse, in collaboration with a shoemaker, an orthotist or prosthetist
Level 3	A level 2 foot centre specialising in
	diabetic foot care, with multiple experts from several disciplines each specialising in this field working together, and acting as a centre of tertiary benchmark

VII.CONCLUSION

Diabetes is becoming a veritable pandemic. Diabetic foot ulcers represent an increasingly important public health problem. Prevention is the only way to reduce the frequency of ulcers, amputations and the cost of diabetic foot disease. They can only be treated within a multidisciplinary framework. Algeria needs to equip itself with appropriate facilities, in particular specialised centres with all the technical resources needed to treat these ulcers. A guide to good medical practice should help to harmonise care across the country and ensure that patients receive better care.The role of the orthopaedic surgeon is central in order to reason in terms of biomechanics to avoid, after conservative or surgical treatment, the creation or persistence of areas of hyper-pressure, which are factors in the recurrence of ulceration. The diabetic foot is a high-risk foot, both neuropathic and vascular. A vascular assessment should always be carried out before considering orthopaedic surgery. If the vascular condition is inadequate, revascularisation procedures should precede any orthopaedic surgery.

VIII. BIBLIOGRAPHY

1. International Diabetes Federation (IDF). https://idf.org/fr/about-diabetes/diabetes-facts-figures/. Accessed on 8 December 2019.

2. J.E. Shaw, R.A. Sicree, P.Z. Zimmet, Global estimates of the prevalence of diabetes for 2010 and 2030. Diabetes Atlas, Published on line 6 November 2009.

3. Bowler PG, Duerden BI, Armstrong DG. Wound microbiology and associated approaches to wound management. ClinMicrobiol Rev 2001; 14: 244-69.

4. Boucher A, Cuiller J. Anatomie topographique descriptive et fonctionnelle page (1625-1718).

5. Jeffcoate WJ, Vileikyte L, Boyko EJ, Armstrong DG, Boulton AJM. Current challenges and opportunities in the prevention and management of diabetic foot ulcers. Diabetes Care 2018; 41: 645-652.

6. Skrepnek GH, Mills JL, Lavery LA, Armstrong DG. Health care service and outcomes among an estimated 6.7 million ambulatory care diabetic foot cases in the U.S. Diabetes Care 2017:40:936-942.

7. Lipsky BA, Peters EJG, Senneville E et al. Expert opinion on the management of of infections of the foot infections. DiabetesMetabResRev. 2012; 28: 163-178.

8. Andrew J.M. Boulton, David G. Armstrong, Robert S. Kirsner, Christopher E. Attinger, Lawrence A. Lavery, Benjamin A. Lipsky, Joseph L. Mills, John S. Steinberg. Diagnosis and Management of Diabetic Foot Complications. 2018 by the American Diabetes Association, Inc.

9. Armstrong DG, Boulton AJM, Bus SA. Diabetic foot ulcers and their recurrence. N Engl J Med 2017;376:2367-2375.

10. Khan T, Armstrong DG. Ulcer-free, hospital-free and activity-rich days: three key metrics for the diabetic foot in remission. JWound Care 2018;27(Suppl. 4):S3-S4.

11. Boghossian J, Miller J, Armstrong D. Offloading the diabetic foot: toward healing wounds and extending ulcer-free days in remission. Chronic Wound Care Management and Research 2017; 4:83-88.

12. Wang A, Xu Z, Mu Y, Ji L. Clinical characteristics and medical costs in patients with diabetic amputation and nondiabetic patients with nonacute amputation in central urban hospitals in China. Int J Low Extrem Wounds. 2014;13:17-21.

13. American Diabetes A. Economic costs of diabetes in the U.S. in 2017. Diabetes Care. 2018;41: 917-28.

14. Krans HMJ, Porta M, Keen H, Staehr-Johansen K, eds. Diabetes care and

research in Europe: the St-Vincent declaration action programme implementation document. 2nd ed. Copenhagen: WHO; 1995.

15. Besse JL, Kawchagie M, Michon P, Ducottet X, Moyen B, Orgiazzi J. Medical surgical team work for diabetic foot management at Lyon-Sud Hospital. Organization and results (Euroforum on the diabetic foot). 4 th Congress of EFFORT (European Federation of National Associations of Orthopaedics and Traumatology), Brussels, Belgium, 1999.

16. French Microbiology Society. The infected diabetic foot. In : REMIC : Société Française de Microbiologie Ed ; 2018 : p.321-328.

17. Denis F, Ploy MC, Martin C, Cattoir V. Cutaneous infections. In: Bactériologie Médicale. Techniques usuelles. Elsevier Masson 3ème edition; 2016: p. 183-193.

18. Besse JL, Michon P, Ducottet X, Lerat JL, Orgiazzi J. Diabetic foot ulcers with osteitis, cellulites or necrosis, treated by orthopaedic surgery: results and interest of preoperative bacteriology and imaging investigations. DFSG International Meeting (Diabetic Foot Study Group), Crieff, Scotland, 2001.

19. Armstrong DG, Peters EJ, Athanasiou KA, Lavery LA. Is there a critical level of plantar foot pressure to identify patients at risk for neuropathic foot ulceration? J Foot Ankle Surg 1998; 37: 303 - 7.

20. Veves A, Van Ross ER, Boulton AJ. Foot pressure measurements in diabetic and nondiabetic amputees. Diabetes Care 1992; 15: 905 - 7.

21. Lavery LA, Lavery DC, Quebedeaux-Farnham TL. Increased foot pressures after great toe amputation in diabetes. Diabete Care 1995; 18: 1640 - 2.

22. Patel GV, Wieman TJ. Effect of metatarsal head resection for diabetic foot ulcers on the dynamic plantar pressure distribution. Am J Surg 1994; 167: 297-301.

23. Nicolaas C. Schaper, Jaap J. van Netten, Jan Apelqvist, Sicco A. Bus, Robert J. Hinchliffe, Benjamin A. Guidelines on the Prevention and Management of Diabetic Foot Disease. Lipskyon behalf of the International Working Group on the Diabetic Foot (IWGDF) Part of the 2019 IWGDF.

24. Malgrange D, Richard JL, Leymarie F, GFPD (Groupe français pied diabétique). Screening diabetic patients at risk for foot ulceration. A multi-centre hospital-based study in France. Diabetes Metab 2003; 29: 261 - 8.

25. Monteiro-Soares M, Boyko EJ, Jeffcoate W, et al. Diabetic foot ulcer classifications: A critical review. Diabetes Metab Res Rev. 2020;36(S1): e3272.

26. Boyko EJ, Seelig AD, Ahroni JH. Limb-and person-level risk factors for lower-limb amputation in the prospective seattle diabetic foot study. Diabetes Care. 2018;41:891-898.

27. Yotsu RR, Pham NM, Oe M, et al. Comparison of characteristics and healing course of diabetic foot ulcers by etiological classification: neuropathic, ischemic, and neuro-ischemic type. J Diabetes Complications. 2014;28(4):528-535.

28. NHS. National diabetes foot care audit third annual report. In: Partnership HQI,editor.https://www.hqip.org.uk/wp-content/uploads/ 2018/03/National-Diabetes-Foot-Care-Audit-2014-2017.pdf; 2018.

29. Oyibo S, Jude E, Tarawneh I, et al. The effects of ulcer size and site, patient's age, sex and type and duration of diabetes on the outcome of diabetic foot ulcers. Diabet Med. 2001;18(2):133-138.

30. Abbas Z, Lutale J, Game F, Jeffcoate W. Comparison of four systems of classification of diabetic foot ulcers in Tanzania. Diabet Med. 2008; 25(2):134-137.

31. Monteiro-Soares M, Martins-Mendes D, Vaz-Carneiro A, DinisRibeiro

M. Lower-limb amputation following foot ulcers in patients with diabetes: classification systems, external validation and comparative analysis. Diabetes Metab Res Rev. 2015;31(5):515-529.

32. Parisi MCR, Zantut-Wittmann DE, Pavin EJ, Machado H, Nery M, Jeffcoate WJ. Comparison of three systems of classification in predicting the outcome of diabetic foot ulcers in a Brazilian population. Eur J Endocrinol. 2008;159 (4):417-422.

33. Ince P, Abbas ZG, Lutale JK, et al. Use of the SINBAD classification system and score in comparing outcome of foot ulcer management on three continents. Diabetes Care. 2008; 31(5):964-967.

34. Bravo-Molina A, Linares-Palomino JP, Vera-Arroyo B, Salmerón-Febres LM, Ros-Díe E. Inter-observer agreement of the Wagner, University of Texas and PEDIS classification systems for the diabetic footsyndrome. Foot Ankle Surg. 2018;24(1):60-64.

35. Forsythe RO, Ozdemir BA, Chemla ES, Jones KG, Hinchliffe RJ. Interobserver reliability of three validated scoring systems in the assessment of diabetic foot ulcers. Int J Low Extrem Wounds. 2016;15(3):213-219.

36. Hicks CW, Canner JK, Karagozlu H, et al. The Society for Vascular Surgery Wound, Ischemia, and foot Infection (WIfI) classification system correlates with cost of care for diabetic foot ulcers treated in a multidisciplinary setting. J Vasc Surg. 2018;67(5):1455-1462.

37. Weaver ML, Hicks CW, Canner JK, et al. The Society for Vascular Surgery Wound, Ischemia, and foot Infection (WIfI) classification system predicts

wound healing better than direct angiosome perfusion in diabetic foot wounds. J Vasc Surg. 2018;68:1473-1481.

38. Wagner FW Jr. The dysvascular foot: a system for diagnosis and treatment. Foot Ankle 1981; 2: 64 -122.

39. International Working Group on the Diabetic Foot. International consensus on the diabetic foot. 1999. Part of the 2019 IWGDF Guidelines on the Prevention and Management of Diabetic Foot Disease, 2019.

40. Chuan F, Tang K, Jiang P, Zhou B, He X. Reliability and validity of the perfusion, extent, depth, infection and sensation (PEDIS) classification system and score in patients with diabetic foot ulcer. PLoS One. 2015; 10(4):e0124739

41. Schaper NC. Diabetic foot ulcer classification system for research purposes: a progress report on criteria for including patients in research studies. Diabetes Metab Res Rev 2004; 20(suppl 1): S90 - 5.

42. Lavery LA, Armstrong DG, Murdoch DP, Peters EJ, Lipsky BA. Validation of the Infectious Diseases Society of America's diabetic foot infection classification system. Clin Infect Dis. 2007;44(4): 562-565.

43. Mills JL, Conte MS, Armstrong DG, Pomposelli F, Schanzer A, Sidawy AN, Andros G. The society for vascular surgery lower extremity threatened limb classification system: Risk stratification based on Wound, Ischemia and foot Infection (WIfI). J Vasc Surg. January 2014; 59:220- 234.

44. Jeon BJ, Choi HJ, Kang JS, Tak MS, Park ES. Comparison of five systems of classification of diabetic foot ulcers and predictive factors for amputation. Int Wound J. 2017;14(3):537-545.

45. Huang Y, Xie T, Cao Y, et al. Comparison of two classification systems in predicting the outcome of diabetic foot ulcers: the Wagner grade and the Saint Elian Wound score systems. Wound Repair Regen. 2015; 23(3):379-385.

46. Frykberg RG, Gordon IL, Reyzelman AM, et al. Feasibility and efficacy of a smart mat technology to predict development of diabetic plantar ulcers. Diabetes Care 2017;40:973-980.

47. Najafi B, Ron E, Enriquez A, Marin I, Razjouyan J, Armstrong DG. Smarter sole survival: will neuropathic patients at high risk for ulceration use a smart insole-based foot protection system? J Diabetes SciTechnol 2017;11:702-713

48. Collins R , Cranny G , Burch J , Aguiar-Ibáñez R , Craig D , Wright K , et al . A systemic review of duplex ultrasound, magnetic resonance angiography and computed tomography angiography for the diagnosis and assessment of symptomatic, lower limb peripheral arterial disease. Health Technol Assess 2007; 11: 1 - 184.

49. Perazella MA. Current status of gadolinium toxicity in patients with kidney

disease. Clin J Am SocNephrol 2009; 4: 461-9.

50. Besse JL, Michon P, Kawchagie M, Ducotter X, Moyen B, Orgiazzi J. Diabetic perforating injuries with osteitis, cellulitis or necrosis, treated by orthopaedic surgery. RevChirOrthop2002; 88 (suppl 6): 2S5.

51. Enderle MD, Coerper S, Schweizer HP, Kopp AF, Thelen MH, Meisner C, et al. Correlation of imaging techniques to histopathology in patients with diabetic foot syndrome and clinical suspicion of chronic osteomyelitis. Diabetes Care 1999; 221: 294 - 9.

52. Delly DM, Schweutzer ME. MR imaging of bone marrow disorders. RadiolClin North Am 1997; 35: 193 - 201.

53. Poirier JY, Garin E, Derrien C, Devillers A, Moisan A, Bourguet P et al. Diagnosis of osteomyelitis in the diabetic foot with a 99mTc-HMPAO leucocyte scintigraphy combined with a 99mTc-MDP bone scintigraphy. Diabetes Metab 2002; 28: 485 - 90.

54. Prompers L, Huijberts M, Apelqvist J, Jude E ,Piaggesi A,n Bakker K et al. Delivery of care to diabetic patients with foot ulcers in daily practice: results of the Eurodiale Study, a prospective cohort study. Diabet Med 2008; 25: 700 - 7.

55. Bayley TS, Yu HM, Rayfield EJ. Patterns of foot examination in a diabetes clinic. Am J Med 1985; 78: 371 - 4.

56. Payne TH, Gabella BA, Michael SL, Young WF, Pickard J, Hofeldt FD et al. Preventive care in diabetes mellitus: current pratices in an urban health-care system. Diabetes Care 1989; 12: 745 - 7.

57. Van Acker K, Oleen-Burkey M, De Decker L, VanmaeleR,VanSchil P, Matricali G, et al. Cost and resource utilization for prevention and treatment of foot lesions in a diabetic foot clinic in Belgium . Diabetes Res ClinPract 2000; 50: 87 - 95.

58. Van Acker K, Vandeleene B, Vermassen F, Leemrijse T. Management of the diabetic foot in a specialised centre. Albe De Coker; 2008.

59. Bus SA, Lavery LA, Monteiro-Soares M, Rasmussen A, Raspovic A, Sacco ICN, Van Netten JJ, on behalf of the International Working Group on the Diabetic Foot (IWGDF). IWGDF guideline on the prevention of foot ulcers in persons with diabetes. Diabetes Metab. Res. Rev. 2019; in press.

60. Bus SA, Armstrong DG, Gooday C; Jarl G; Caravaggi CF, Viswanathan V; Lazzarini PA; on behalf of the International Working Group on the Diabetic Foot (IWGDF). IWGDF Guideline on offloading foot ulcers in persons with diabetes. Diabetes Metab.Res.Rev. 2019; in press.

61. Hinchliffe RJ, Forsythe R, Apelqvist J, Boyko EJ, Fitridge R, Hong JP, et al. IWGDF Guideline on diagnosis, prognosis and management of peripheral artery

disease in patients with a foot ulcer and diabetes. Diabetes Metab. Res. Rev. 2019; in press.

62. Lipsky BA, Senneville , Abbas Z, Aragón-Sánchez J, Diggle M, Embil J, et al. IWGDF Guideline on the diagnosis and treatment of foot infection in persons with diabetes. Diabetes Metab. Res. Rev. 2019; in press.

63. Rayman G, Vas P, Dhatariya K, Driver V, Hartemann A, Londahl M, et al. IWGDF Guideline on interventions to enhance healing of foot ulcers in persons with diabetes. Diabetes Metab. Res. Rev. 2019; in press.

64. Monteiro-Soares M, Russell D, Boyko EJ, Jeffcoate W, Mills JL, Morbach S, Game F. IWGDF Guidelines on the classification of diabetic foot ulcers. Diabetes Metab. Res. Rev. 2019; in press.

65. Leibner ED, Brodsky JW, Pollo FE, Baum BS, Edmonds BW. Unloading mechanism in the total contact cast. Foot Ankle Int 2006; 27: 281 - 5.

66. Ali R, Qureshi A, Yaqoob MY, Shakil M. Total contact cast for neuropathic diabetic foot ulcers. J Coll Physicians Surg Pak 2008; 18: 695 - 8.

67. Dhalla R, Johnson JE, Engsberg J. Can the use of a terminal device augment plantar pressure reduction with a total contact cast? Foot Ankle Int 2003; 24: 500 - 5.

68. Guyton GP. An analysis of iatrogenic complications from the total contact cast. Foot Ankle Int 2005; 26: 903 - 7.

69. Beuker BJ, van Deursen RW, Price P, Manning EA, Van Baal JG, Harding KG. Plantar pressure in off-loading devices used in diabetic ulcer treatment. Wound Repair Regen 2005; 13: 537 - 42.

70. DiLiberto FE, Baumhauer JF, Wilding GE, Nawoczenski DA. Alterations in plantar pressure with different walking boot designs. Foot Ankle Int 2007; 28: 55 - 60.

71. Caravaggi C, Faglia E, De Giglio R, Montero M, Quarantiello A, Sommariva E et al. Effectiveness and safety of a non-removable fiberglass off-bearing cast versus a therapeutic shoe in the treatment of neuropathic ulcers. A randomized study. Diabetes Care 2000; 23: 1746 - 51.

72. Wu SC, Jensen JL, Weber AK, Robinson DE, Armstrong DG. Use of pressure offloading devices in diabetic foot ulcers: do we practice what we preach? Diabetes Care 2008; 31: 2118 - 9.

73. Laborde JM. Neuropathic plantar forefoot ulcers treated with tendon lengthenings. Foot Ankle Int 2008; 29: 378 - 84.

74. Mueller MJ, Sinacore DR, Hastings MK, Strube MJ, Johnson JE. Effect of Achilles tendon lengthening on neuropathic plantar ulcers. A randomized clinical trial. J Bone Joint Surg (Am)2003; 85: 1436 - 45.

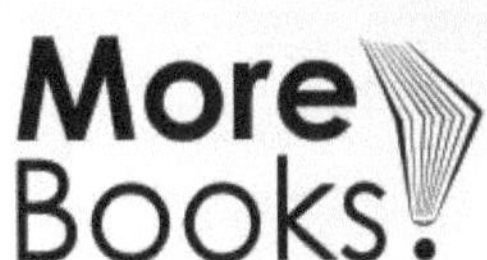

More
Books!

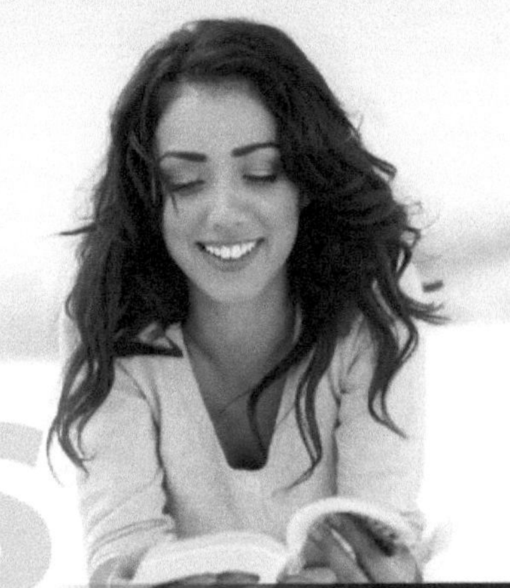

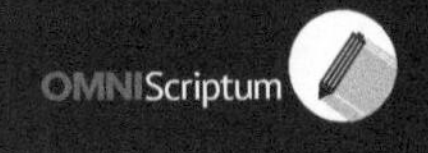

info@omniscriptum.com
www.omniscriptum.com
OMNIScriptum

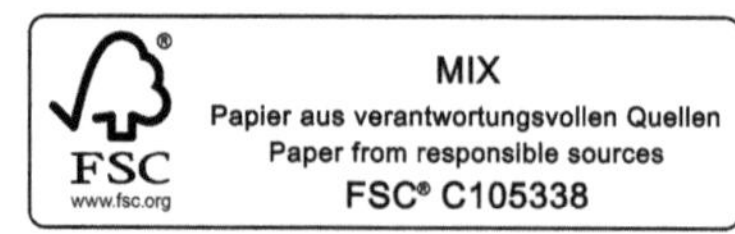

Printed by Books on Demand GmbH, Norderstedt / Germany